Self Assessment Manual

2

Oral Medicine and Diagnosis

BERTRAM COHEN DDS, MSD, FDSRCS, FRCPath
*Nuffield Professor, Director of Department of Dental Science,
Royal College of Surgeons of England*

DAVID K MASON BDS, MD, FDSRCS, FRCPath
Professor of Oral Medicine, University of Glasgow

and

DAVID E POSWILLO DDS, DSc, FDSRCS, MRCPath
*Professor of Oral Surgery and Pathology, University of Adelaide,
South Australia*

WILLIAM HEINEMANN MEDICAL BOOKS LTD
London

First published 1978
© B. Cohen, D. K. Mason and D. E. Poswillo 1978

ISBN 0 433 06193 6

Printed in Great Britain by Wood Westworth & Co. Ltd.,
Park Road, St. Helens, Merseyside

PREFACE

This book includes material collected over many years from many different hospitals and from many different colleagues. Because the source is so difficult to trace in every instance we would like to resort to a blanket acknowledgment by collectively thanking those who provided illustrations included in this compilation. More specifically we owe our thanks to Mr. P. Broadbery of the Medical Illustration Unit at the Queen Victoria Hospital, East Grinstead, for his photographic skills and to Miss Carole Meadows, Mrs. Isabel McGuire, and Mrs. Audrey Orme for their secretarial assistance. Finally we are grateful to Mr. R. Emery and Mr. C. Jarvis of Heinemann for their help in the genesis and development of this book.

We have adopted the format of questions and answers based on illustrations to overcome some of the difficulties of revision and continuing education for busy dental practitioners and those who are preparing for higher examinations. There is no possibility of covering the field comprehensively in a book of this size. We have chosen to include both the commonplace and the extraordinary with a view to providing revision, information, and above all, stimulation. We are aware that in some instances the pictures shown are neither sufficiently typical nor, indeed, sufficiently fine in detail to permit recognition by even the most experienced diagnostician. Nevertheless we feel that the wording of the questions will often stimulate thought; the answers, we hope, may then encourage a broader approach to diagnosis and management in addition to providing an impetus to further enquiry from the literature. Above all the demonstration that so many clinical appearances are of a non-specific nature should serve to emphasise the need for taking a thorough history and making a careful clinical examination before diagnosis is attempted.

Our format differs from that which is customary in Multiple Choice Questions, and had this book been intended merely as preparation for examinations it would have been necessary to reduce the length of our questions and to curtail the answers considerably. This however, would have greatly reduced the value of the book for self-assessment as distinct from examiner-assessment. We decided that its usefulness would be enhanced rather than diminished by our exceeding the limited time available for the staccato questions and answers inseparable from the MCQ formula.

Finally we must anticipate the possibility of being taken to task for occasional glimpses of levity in our text. This is not unintentional. In compiling SAM I and SAM II we found that we had not only learned a lot from one another but also that we had enjoyed ourselves in the process; we can only hope that our readers may feel the same way.

B. Cohen
D. K. Mason
D. E. Poswillo

Note: When referring to eponymously designated syndromes we have followed the recommendation set out in **The Lancet** (1975, i, 513) that the possessive form be discontinued.

QUESTION SECTION

PLATE 1

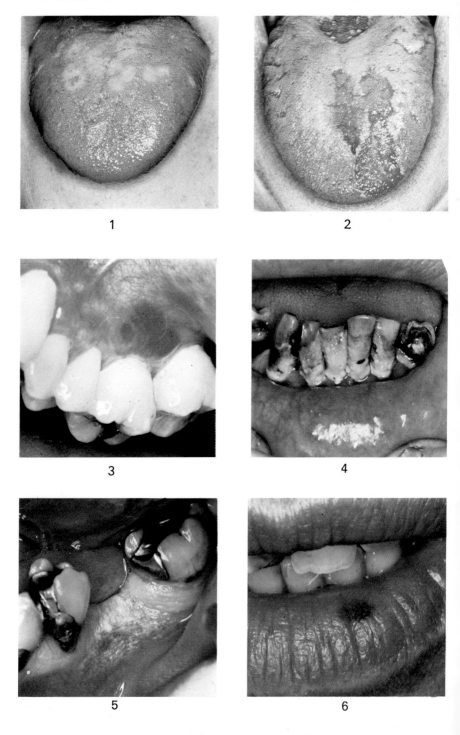

1

2

3

4

5

6

PLATE 1

1. (a) What is this condition?
   (b) What further clinical examinations are required apart from the oral examination?
   (c) What further laboratory examinations are required?

2. (a) Lesions of this type become increasingly severe/less severe with age.
   (b) This is/is not a familial condition.
   (c) The lesion can/cannot be eliminated by antibiotic therapy.
   (d) The lesion is likely/unlikely to show histological signs of premalignancy?
   (e) What is this condition?

3. Male aged 65 years with a history of oral blisters and ulcers for past six months
   (a) What oral abnormality is shown?
   (b) What could be the disease of which this change is typical?
   (c) What other investigations would help to establish the diagnosis?
   (d) What is the treatment of this condition?

4. This patient has been seriously ill with abdominal pain and limb weakness and also has sialorrhoea.
   (a) What abnormalities do you observe?
   (b) What could be the underlying condition?
   (c) What other clinical manifestations occur?
   (d) Which of the following occupations could have contributed to this condition: (i) dentist (ii) dental nurse (iii) smelter (iv) fisherman (v) miner (vi) prostitute (vii) welder?

5. This patient has a bilateral facial rash.
   (a) What abnormality is present on the oral mucosa?
   (b) What is the likely diagnosis?
   (c) What are the microscopic appearances?
   (d) What treatment is called for?

6. (a) What are the cells containing pigment in this lesion?
   (b) Are they originally derived from the neural crest/basal epithelium/the retinal anlage?
   (c) Are these cells most numerous in dark-skinned races?
   (d) What is the commonest reason for pigmentation of oral tissues?

Answers on page 52–53

PLATE 2

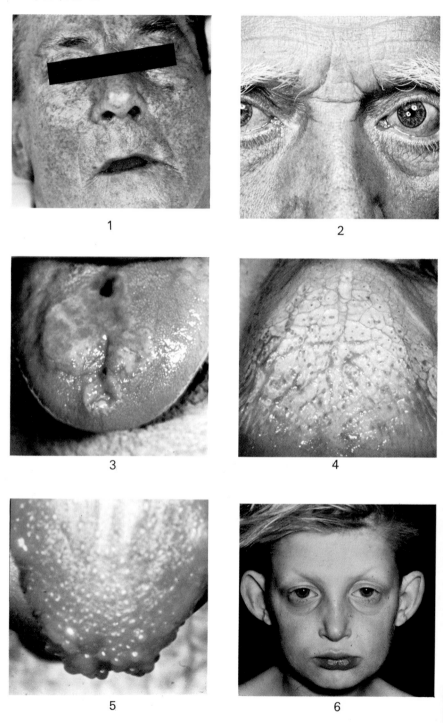

1

2

3

4

5

6

PLATE 2

1. (a) What serious disease should be suspected?
   (b) Of what significance would this be with regard to dental treatment?
   (c) Is the patient likely to be (i) athletic (ii) alcoholic (iii) ascitic (iv) anaemic?

2. (a) What is this condition?
   (b) What is the cause of the discolouration?
   (c) Into what 3 main types can this disorder be classified?
   (d) Of what dental significance is this condition?

3. In addition to the lesions illustrated the gingivae are swollen and bleeding.
   (a) What systemic disease should be suspected?
   (b) Why should the tongue be swollen and ulcerated?
   (c) Why should the gingivae be swollen and bleeding?
   (d) What are the principles of management of the oral manifestations of this condition?

4. (a) What is this condition in the palate of a middle-aged male?
   (b) What is the reason for the irregularity of the surface?
   (c) Is this a premalignant condition?
   (d) What is the treatment?

5. (a) Of what clinical syndrome could this be an oral manifestation?
   (b) How would you confirm your diagnosis?
   (c) What is the prognosis?
   (d) What other tumour is known to be associated with this condition?

6. (a) What dental defects would you expect to find in this child?
   (b) Is the condition likely to be found in other members of the family and if so, which?
   (c) What facial features suggest the diagnosis of this condition?

Answers on page 53–54

PLATE 3

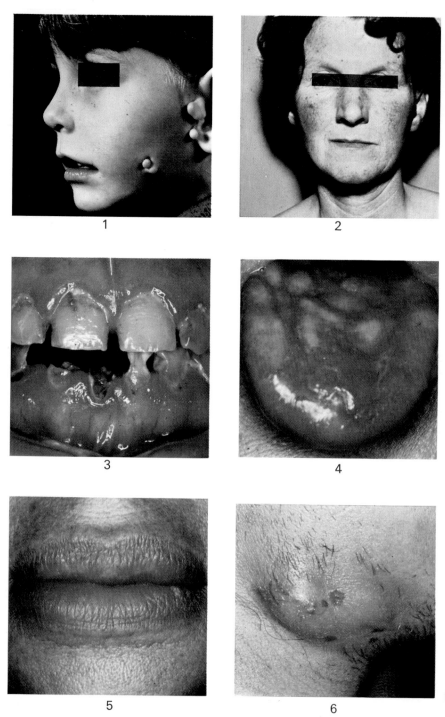

PLATE 3

1. **(a)** What are these facial appendages?
   (b) In which of the following syndromes may they be commonly found: Goldenhar, unilateral facial necrosis, otomandibular dysostosis, hemifacial microsomia and microtia, lateral facial dysplasia, first arch syndrome?

2. **(a)** What serious disease could be suspected from the facial appearance?
   (b) Of what significance could this be in regard to dental surgical treatment?

3. Dental health was good until one year ago.
   (a) What investigations would you wish to carry out?
   (b) What treatment could be suggested?

4. This patient aged 72 years has chronic renal failure with uraemia.
   (a) What oral abnormality is present?
   (b) What other oral symptoms or signs may occur in this condition?
   (c) Are oral manifestations common?
   (d) How might this condition be treated?

5. There has been a gradual, progressive enlargement of lips and lower jaw.
   (a) What endocrine disorder could produce this appearance and what is it due to?
   (b) What other manifestations of this disease occur?
   (c) What complications may occur?
   (d) What investigations are necessary to establish a diagnosis?
   (e) How is this condition treated?

6. This patient had a swelling of long standing at the angle of the jaw.
   (a) What specific chronic infection may occur in this area and produce multiple sinuses?
   (b) What is the causative organism?
   (c) How would you confirm your diagnosis?
   (d) Where else in the body might this specific chronic infection occur?
   (e) How would you treat this condition?

Answers on pages 55-6

PLATE 4

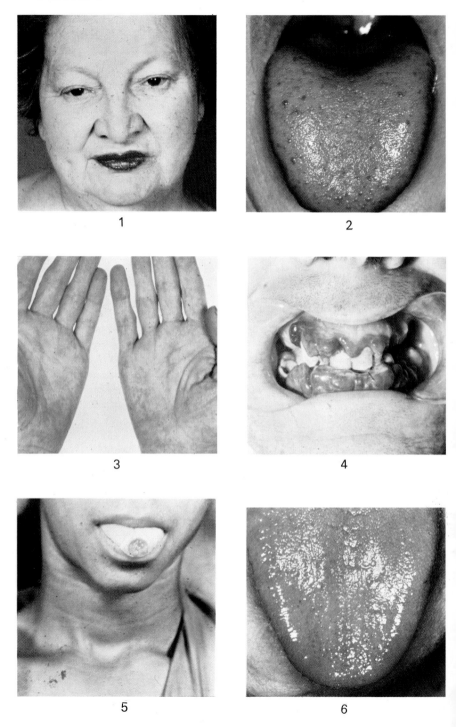

1

2

3

4

5

6

PLATE 4

1. This 60-year-old lady complains of tiredness and has developed generalised swelling of her face.
   (a) What clinical state is shown here?
   (b) What is the cause of this appearance?
   (c) Of what significance could this be with regard to dental treatment?

2. (a) What clinical abnormality is demonstrated here?
   (b) What is the name of this condition?
   (c) Is it hereditary/inflammatory/neoplastic/venereal in origin?
   (d) What sites are usually affected?
   (e) What complications may occur?
   (f) Is there any effective local treatment?

3. (a) What abnormality is present on this patient's hands?
   (b) What precautions might be necessary when dental treatment is carried out?

4. This malnourished patient complained of severe pain in his knee joints and bleeding in the mouth. Extensive bruising of the skin was evident, several joints were swollen, and his teeth were loose.
   (a) What dietary deficiency is likely to be present?
   (b) In what circumstances was this first reported?
   (c) In what population groups is it most likely to occur today?
   (d) What are the histological appearances of an oral lesion?

5. This lesion was present for three weeks in a female aged 18 years.
   (a) How would you confirm a diagnosis of (i) squamous cell carcinoma (ii) strawberry tongue (iii) syphilis (iv) trauma?

   (b) In what order would you exclude these possibilities?

6. This patient complains of a burning tongue. Blood examination revealed the following: Haemoglobin 8.5 g/100 ml, Mean Corpuscular Volume — low, and Mean Corpuscular Haemoglobin — low.
   (a) What is the condition seen in the tongue?
   (b) Of what generalized haematological disorder could it be indicative?
   (c) What further laboratory findings would provide confirmation?
   (d) How would you treat this patient?

Answers on page 56−57

PLATE 5

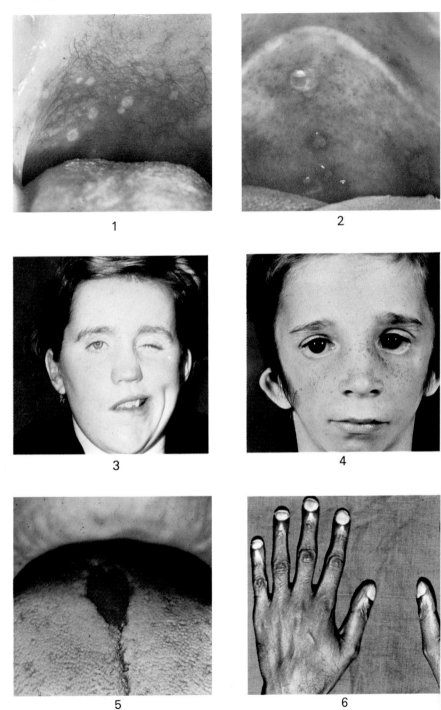

1

2

3

4

5

6

PLATE 5

1. This lesion suddenly appeared in this child's mouth along with sore throat and fever.
   (a) What oral lesion is demonstrated here?
   (b) What differential diagnoses would you consider?
   (c) How would you investigate this patient further?
   (d) What treatment might be required?

2. (a) What is the abnormality on the soft palate behind the post-dam of the denture?
   (b) What investigation would you carry out immediately?
   (c) What serological examination would be indicated?
   (d) What other areas of the body might be affected?

3. This patient has been asked to show her teeth.
   (a) What abnormality is apparent?
   (b) What other name is often used for this condition when the lower motor neurone is affected?
   (c) In what syndromes can this condition be a feature?
   (d) Which of the following are proven causative factors in this condition: **(i)** smoking **(ii)** lack of fresh vegetables in the diet **(iii)** pollution **(iv)** sudden changes in temperature?

4. (a) What facial characteristics indicate the specific syndrome affecting this child?
   (b) What is the most common dental defect?

5. (a) This is/is not a developmental defect.
   (b) What theory has been proposed for a developmental origin?
   (c) What alternative to a developmental origin has been put forward?
   (d) This lesion is/is not commonly premalignant?

6. (a) What is the abnormality shown here?
   (b) In which of the following does it commonly occur: **(i)** port drinkers **(ii)** chimney sweeps **(iii)** glass blowers **(iv)** bronchiectasis **(v)** manicurists **(vi)** congenital heart disease?
   (c) What is the clinical significance of the observation?

Answers on page 58 −59

PLATE 6

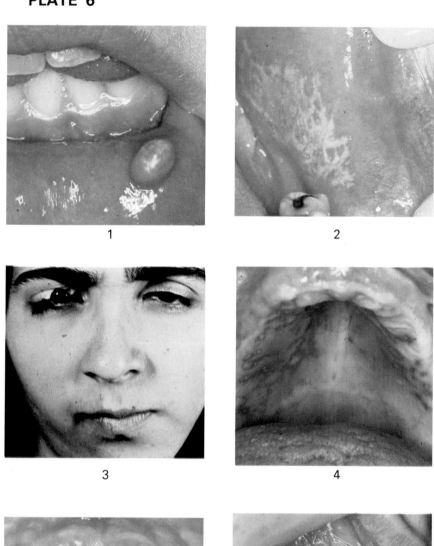

1

2

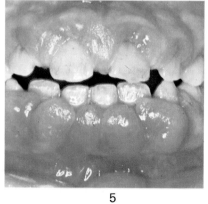

3

4

5

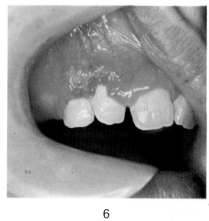

6

PLATE 6

1. Swelling of lip intermittently for three months.
   (a) What is this condition likely to be?
   (b) Is this a common site? Where else may it occur?
   (c) Enumerate three histological appearances of significance?
   (d) What is the likeliest cause of this condition?

2. (a) What is this lesion and what is the morphological variant?
   (b) Name three other morphological variants.
   (c) What is the sex ratio?

3. (a) Which of these jaw defects is likely to accompany the
       obvious malformation shown: Open bite, jaw-winking
       syndrome, missing lateral incisors, condylar hypoplasia,
       unilateral condylar hyperplasia, pathological fracture?

4. This type of oral infection due to herpes simplex is common in
   infants and children but unusual, as shown here, in a patient
   aged 60 years and edentulous.
   (a) What is the oral abnormality demonstrated?
   (b) In what special circumstances (as in this case) might it
       occur?

5. (a) What is this abnormality?
   (b) What drug could cause this appearance?
   (c) Why is it used?
   (d) What is the nature of the oral lesions?
   (e) What are the principles of treatment?

6. This lesion of the gingivae and oral mucosa did not respond to
   treatment. The patient has had a cough for many weeks and has
   lost weight. Some months ago he developed raised, tender,
   erythematous lesions of the skin overlying both shins. He
   complains of sweating during sleep.
   (a) What is the diagnosis and how would you confirm it?
   (b) What other part of the body would you examine?
   (c) How would you treat this condition?

Answers on page 59

PLATE 7

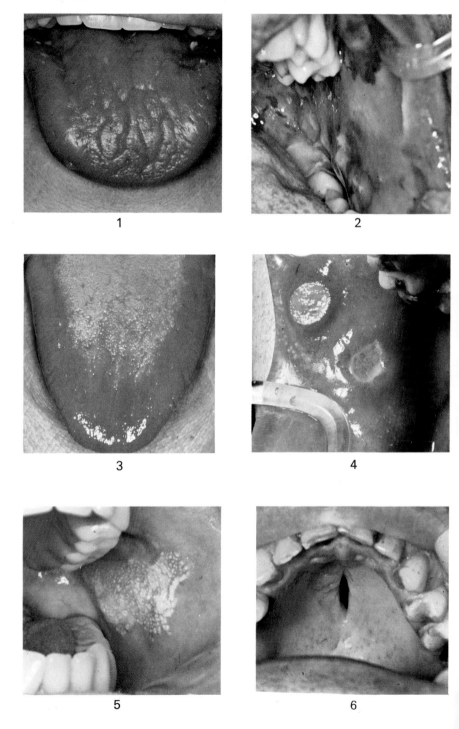

1

2

3

4

5

6

PLATE 7

1. History of xerostomia for 3 years.
   (a) What abnormal appearances are evident?
   (b) What other parts of the body may also be affected?
   (c) How would you investigate the mouth dryness?
   (d) What other laboratory tests should be carried out?

2. Oral lesions in an 18-year-old girl. She also had some cervical lymphadenopathy.
   (a) What is the condition?
   (b) What could be the cause?
   (c) What investigations would you wish to carry out?

3. Sore tongue for one week. Her general health has been good but 3 weeks ago she had tonsillitis which responded to antibiotics.
   (a) What is the clinical abnormality and how could it have arisen?
   (b) How would you confirm your diagnosis?
   (c) What treatment is indicated?

4. (a) What recurrent oral condition is shown here?
   (b) What other parts of the body could be involved?
   (c) What other investigations would you carry out?
   (d) How would you treat this condition if all the investigations were normal?

5. (a) What is the differential diagnosis?
   (b) What clinical appearance demonstrated here might indicate the possible prognosis?
   (c) What is the first extra-oral clinical examination you would carry out?
   (d) What investigation would you request?

6. This condition has been present in this 55-year-old man for three months.
   (a) What abnormality is present?
   (b) Which disease processes may cause this?
   (c) What investigative procedures would you perform?

Answers on page 60 – 61

PLATE 8

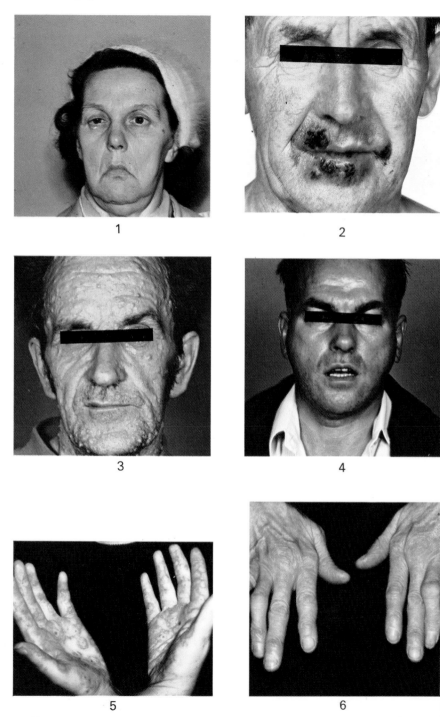

1

2

3

4

5

6

PLATE 8

1. This patient assumes this appearance especially when tired. Occasionally her temporomandibular joints 'stick' and she is unable to masticate for long.
   (a) What disease could cause this condition?
   (b) How can it be diagnosed?
   (c) Can it be treated?
   (d) Can it be cured?

2. (a) What facial abnormalities are shown?
   (b) In the absence of trauma, from what underlying condition could this arise?
   (c) What investigations are required?
   (d) What oral lesions might be present?

3. These multiple swellings developed over the past few years.
   (a) What is this condition likely to be?
   (b) What other skin manifestation may occur?
   (c) Can these swellings occur on the oral mucosa also?
   (d) What complication can occur in this condition?

4. This patient has bilateral parotid enlargement. The swelling is painless and has developed gradually.
   (a) What is this condition called?
   (b) Enumerate three possible causes?
   (c) What is the prognosis?

5. (a) What abnormality is present on the hands of this patient?
   (b) What oral condition may accompany this lesion?
   (c) What is the cause?
   (d) What is the treatment?

6. (a) What is the deformity shown here in a 65-year-old female?
   (b) What oral manifestations might accompany this deformity?
   (c) What other factors would have to be considered when this patient receives dental treatment?

Answers on page 61–62

PLATE 9

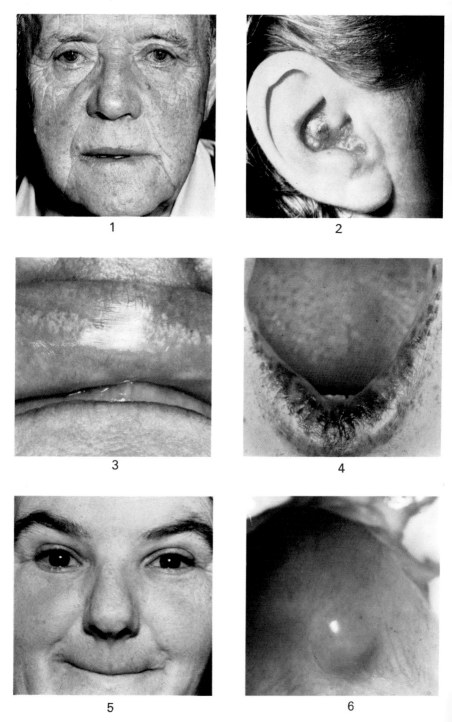

1

2

3

4

5

6

PLATE 9

1. (a) From what blood disease might this patient suffer?
   (b) What is the cause of this condition?
   (c) What are the main features of this disease?
   (d) What dental complications are associated with this condition?

2. In addition to this condition of the external ear, this patient has facial palsy.
   (a) What is the syndrome?
   (b) What is the cause?
   (c) How does this condition differ from shingles?
   (d) What sensory function can be impaired?
   (e) What treatment is indicated and what is the prognosis?

3. (a) What common condition is apparent on this slide? (Ignore the central highlight).
   (b) Is this neoplastic, traumatic, degenerative, or developmental in origin?
   (c) Where else does it occur on the oral mucosa?
   (d) What treatment is required?

4. (a) In what syndrome is this appearance found?
   (b) What other abnormalities may accompany this appearance?
   (c) What clinical complications might arise in this syndrome?
   (d) Where else might pigmentation occur in this condition?

5. There is a history of fractures of the long bones.
   (a) What facial appearance might have made you suspect a disease of bone?
   (b) How does this appearance come about?
   (c) What oral manifestation may be present?
   (d) Can this condition be cured?

6. This swelling had gradually appeared in the palate in a child aged 6 years.
   (a) What are the likeliest diagnoses?
   (b) What clinical investigation could you perform to confirm your diagnosis?
   (c) What treatment is required?

Answers on page 62−63

19

PLATE 10

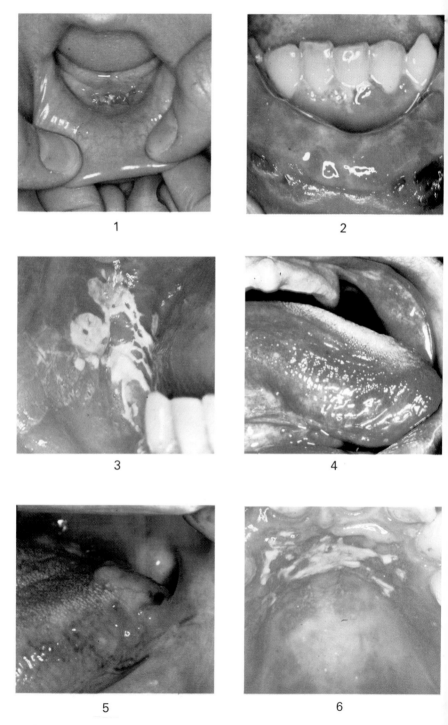

1

2

3

4

5

6

PLATE 10

1. This oral ulcer in a female aged 45 did not heal. Biopsy revealed a giant cell granuloma with Langhans type giant cells and epithelioid cells but no caseation. Parotid salivary glands were enlarged. Lung X-ray showed bilateral hilar lymphadenopathy.
   (a) What is the probable diagnosis?
   (b) What blood examinations would be helpful?
   (c) What skin tests would be helpful?
   (d) What treatment may be necessary?

2. (a) What is this oral appearance usually called?
   (b) What can it be caused by?
   (c) What other manifestations might occur apart from the oral signs?
   (d) What is the treatment?
   (e) Is it likely to recur?

3. The patient complained of roughness of the mucosa for several months.
   (a) What are the three main conditions to be considered in a differential diagnosis?
   (b) How would you reach a definitive diagnosis?
   (c) With which of the following are lesions of this sort associated: (i) Ehlers Danlos syndrome (ii) benign lymphoepithelial lesion (iii) lupus erythematosus (iv) leucocytosis (v) syphilis?

4. A female aged 55 years has had a sore tongue for some weeks. Blood examination showed low haemoglobin — 11 g/100 ml, and macrocytosis.
   (a) What abnormality is demonstrated here?
   (b) What haematological disorder may be present?
   (c) What further examinations are required?
   (d) What neurological complication can develop?

5. (a) What are the spherical structures on the lateral border of the tongue and what abnormality is present?
   (b) What treatment might be helpful in this case?
   (c) What is a common reason for patients with this lesion seeking advice?

6. History of cytotoxic drug therapy.
   (a) What could this lesion on the palate be?
   (b) What investigations might confirm the diagnosis?
   (c) What treatment should be prescribed?

Answers on page 63—64

PLATE 11

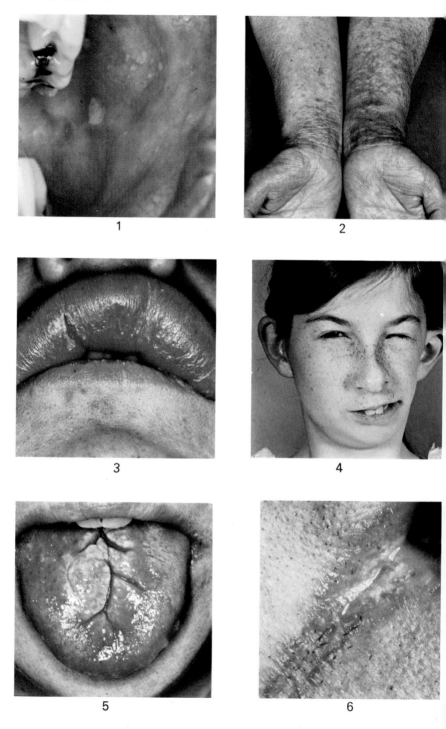

1

2

3

4

5

6

PLATE 11

1. (a) What common recurrent type of oral ulceration occurs in this site and which type is shown here?
   (b) What mucosal developmental abnormality is also shown?
   (c) How would you investigate this patient?
   (d) How would you treat this patient if the investigations were negative?

2. This male aged 45 complains of an itchy rash on his wrist and forearms. He also has felt some discomfort intraorally.
   (a) How would you describe this appearance of skin?
   (b) What is the probable diagnosis?
   (c) What could be the oral manifestations?
   (d) What other tissues apart from skin and mucosa may be affected?
   (e) Are oral lesions always accompanied by skin lesions?

3. (a) What is the term used to describe this persistent firm swelling of the upper lip?
   (b) What could be the cause?
   (c) What treatment should be prescribed?

4. (a) What is this deformity?
   (b) Does this defect arise (i) before birth (ii) during birth (iii) in infancy (iv) in adolescence? How can you be certain?
   (c) How commonly does it occur?
   (d) What is the probable cause?
   (e) How can mandibular contour be restored? When?

5. This is a recurrent infection.
   (a) What is the condition likely to be?
   (b) What could be the cause of such a condition?
   (c) How can it be further investigated?

6. (a) What is this condition?
   (b) What are the common local causes?
   (c) What organisms may be involved?
   (d) Of which is this likely to be an oral manifestation: (i) avitaminosis (ii) oligiasis (iii) measles (iv) psoriasis?

Answers on page 65–66

PLATE 12

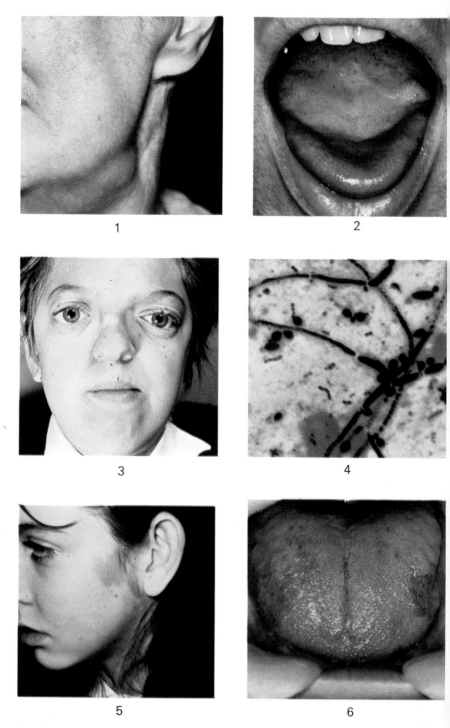

1

2

3

4

5

6

PLATE 12

1. This patient has had Sjogren syndrome for five years. Over the past two months she has developed a new symptom, discernible in the illustration.
   (a) What complication would you suspect?
   (b) In what proportion of patients with Sjogren syndrome might this complication occur?
   (c) How would you confirm your diagnosis?

2. (a) Of what disturbance of salivary function is this an example?
   (b) Is this condition more or less common than xerostomia?
   (c) Name two dental causes.
   (d) Name two systemic diseases associated with this condition.

3. (a) Which of the following oral conditions may be associated with this facial appearance: Open bite, condylar aplasia, high arched palate, severe malocclusion, bifid tongue?
   (b) What is the greatest risk to health in early childhood?

4. (a) What organism is demonstrated on this Gram-stained smear?
   (b) Can this organism be grown in culture? If so, which medium?
   (c) What oral lesions are associated with this organism?
   (d) What drugs can be used to combat this infection?
   (e) What drugs might initiate it?

5. In addition to the abnormality shown this young girl has a diffuse bony swelling of her maxilla.
   (a) What is a likely diagnosis?
   (b) What other clinical manifestations of this condition would you look for?

6. This patient complains of 'bruising' of her tongue although she was unaware of trauma to these areas. She has also been generally unwell, feeling easily tired for the past few months.
   (a) What serious disease should be suspected?
   (b) What other clinical signs should be sought for?
   (c) What is the pigment?
   (d) How would you investigate this patient?

Answers on page 66–67

PLATE 13

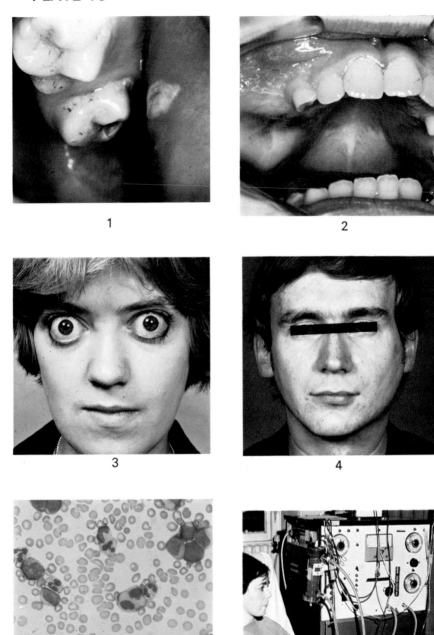

1

2

3

4

5

6

PLATE 13

1. (a) What is the cause of this ulceration?
   (b) What important structure does the ulcer include?
   (c) What treatment would be required?

2. Painless maxillary swelling with no well defined border; girl aged 10 years.
   (a) What is the likely diagnosis?
   (b) How would you seek to confirm your diagnosis?
   (c) How would you treat this condition?
   (d) Of what syndrome might this be a part?

3. (a) What clinical condition is apparent here?
   (b) What is the underlying disease?
   (c) What complications may occur during dental treatment?

4. This patient complains of painful salivary glands.
   (a) What is the probable cause of this common condition?
   (b) What is the infectious agent?
   (c) How is it spread?
   (d) What laboratory test will confirm your diagnosis?
   (e) In a severe case what complications can occur?

5. (a) What abnormality is shown on this peripheral blood film?
   (b) What different types of this condition may occur?
   (c) What are the oral manifestations?
   (d) How often are oral signs and symptoms present?

6. This patient has renal failure and is undergoing haemodialysis.
   (a) To what diseases are these patients particularly susceptible?
   (b) What special factors have to be considered in providing dental treatment for these patients?

Answers on page 68

PLATE 14

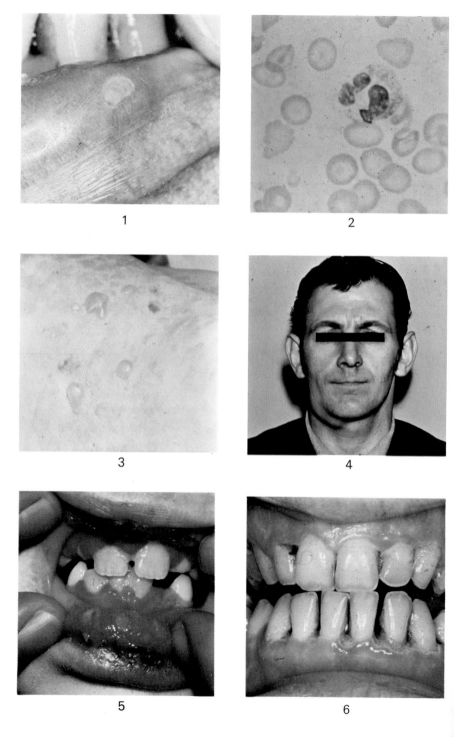

1

2

3

4

5

6

PLATE 14

1. This is a recurrent lesion. Blood investigations demonstrated the following results:

   Iron saturation 10%
   Whole blood folate 40 ug/l
   Serum Vitamin B12 300 ng/ml

   (a) In what way are these results abnormal?
   (b) Of what more general condition may this be the oral manifestation?
   (c) How would you manage such a patient?
   (d) What treatment could be necessary?

2. Blood film taken from a 55-year-old female with a sore tongue and some difficulty in eating and swallowing.
   (a) What abnormal appearances are demonstrated?
   (b) What oral signs could be present in such a patient?
   (c) What syndrome may be associated with this condition?
   (d) How would you investigate?

3. These skin lesions were seen in a patient with a history of oral ulceration.
   (a) What abnormality is shown here?
   (b) What could the diagnosis be? Which condition is most likely?
   (c) How could the diagnosis be confirmed?
   (d) What other internal or systemic disease may be associated with this condition?

4. This patient aged 35 years has painless discrete rubbery swellings of submandibular lymph nodes, gradually enlarging, of two months' duration. He feels unwell and has lost weight.
   (a) What is the likely diagnosis?
   (b) What other clinical signs should be sought for?
   (c) What other radiological examinations are called for?
   (d) How would you confirm your diagnosis?
   (e) What is the prognosis and treatment of this condition?

5. Child aged 7 years.
   (a) What abnormality is shown here?
   (b) What is the probable diagnosis in this age group?
   (c) If it recurs do lesions affect the oral mucosa?
   (d) How could you confirm your diagnosis?
   (e) What treatment would you advise?

6. (a) What is this condition?
   (b) How would you confirm your diagnosis?

Answers on page 69-70

PLATE 15

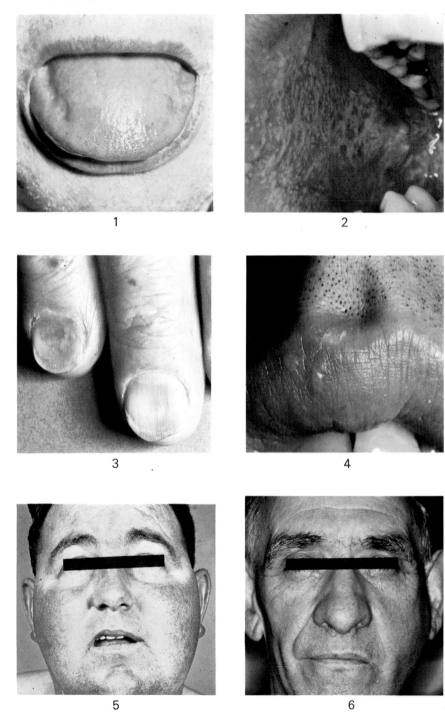

1

2

3

4

5

6

PLATE 15

1. This patient, a male aged 35 years, has multiple myelomatosis.
   (a) What oral abnormality is evident?
   (b) What could be the cause of the abnormality?
   (c) What staining methods would be useful to apply to sections of a biopsy of the tongue?
   (d) What are the principal features supporting the diagnosis of myelomatosis?

2. (a) Of what condition is this an example?
   (b) What other tissues of the body may be affected?
   (c) What is the treatment and prognosis?

3. (a) What is the abnormality demonstrated?
   (b) What is the cause of this condition?
   (c) What is the sex prevalence?
   (d) What other clinical manifestations might occur if this condition is part of a syndrome? What is the syndrome called?

4. This lesion was of sudden onset, preceded by 'a prickly sensation' in the affected area.
   (a) What is the most likely diagnosis?
   (b) What is the cause?
   (c) What is the source of the causative agent?
   (d) What factors may predispose to this condition?
   (e) What empirical treatment might be recommended?

5. Facial appearance has changed during long term systemic drug therapy.
   (a) What drugs could give this appearance?
   (b) For what conditions might these drugs be used?
   (c) What complication affecting dental treatment could occur?
   (d) How might that problem be overcome?

6. This patient has acute pain and pus can be expressed from the parotid duct.
   (a) What circumstances may predispose to this disorder?
   (b) What bacteria are most commonly responsible?
   (c) What treatment would you recommend?
   (d) What investigation is contraindicated in such a case?

Answers on page 70 – 71

PLATE 16

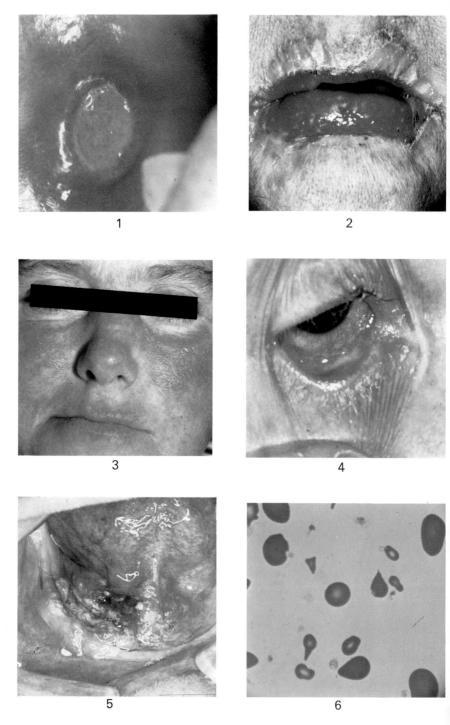

1

2

3

4

5

6

PLATE 16

1. Lesions of this sort appear at about the same time each month in this female subject.
   (a) What type of ulceration is this?
   (b) At what stage in the menstrual cycle does ulceration usually occur?
   (c) At what stage does it usually heal?
   (d) What is the basis of treatment in these patients?

2. This 65-year-old lady has neglected her oral condition for some years.
   (a) Given the results of blood examination were normal, what examinations would you carry out to establish a diagnosis?
   (b) What is the treatment?
   (c) What is the prognosis?

3. (a) What disease is characteristically associated with this type of rash?
   (b) What oral manifestations of this condition can occur?
   (c) What further investigation of the oral mucosal lesions is desirable?

4. This patient has marked conjunctivitis.
   (a) In which syndromes are oral manifestations associated with this appearance of the eyes? Enumerate the oral manifestations of each.

5. (a) What is the probable diagnosis of this enlarging lesion that first appeared three months previously?
   (b) What clinical signs would support the diagnosis?
   (c) What forms of non-surgical treatment are available?

6. This is a blood film from a 50-year-old female.
   (a) What abnormalities are demonstrated?
   (b) What further tests should be carried out?
   (c) Are there any good reasons for thinking that the patient might be (i) malnourished (ii) pregnant (iii) a Finnish fishwife (iv) epileptic?

Answers on page 71 –72

PLATE 17

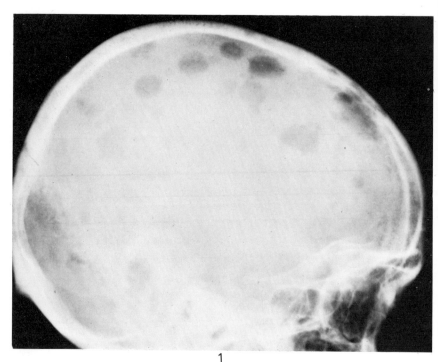

1

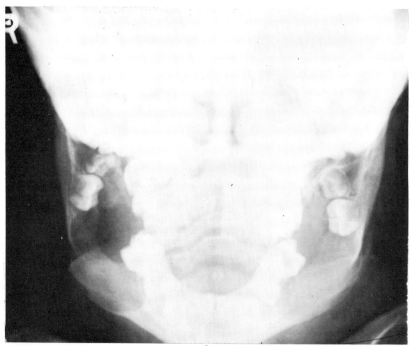

2

PLATE 17

1. (a) What abnormality is shown here?
   (b) What is the differential diagnosis?
   (c) In reaching a definitive diagnosis how would you be
       assisted by **(i)** urinalysis **(ii)** blood chemistry **(iii)**
       examination of bone marrow **(iv)** bacteriological tests **(v)**
       culturing for virus **(vi)** discriminant analysis of multivariate
       positron scans?

2. (a) The radiological abnormalities present are indicative of **(i)**
       Gorlin syndrome **(ii)** Hunter syndrome **(iii)** rickets **(iv)**
       Hurler syndrome **(v)** Morquio Ullrich syndrome. Which?
   (b) Is there a laboratory test that will help to establish the
       differential diagnosis?

Answers on page 73

PLATE 18

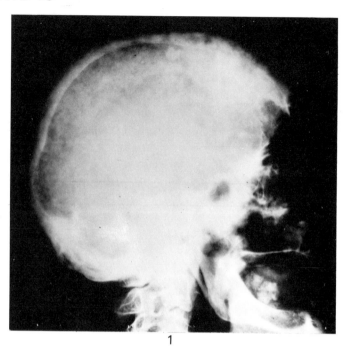

1

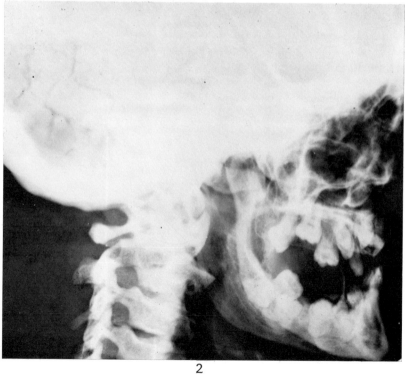

2

PLATE 18

1. This man, aged 65 years, had ill-fitting dentures and hypercementosis of his remaining maxillary teeth.
   (a) What abnormality is shown on this lateral skull X-ray?
   (b) What disease can give these appearances?
   (c) What biochemical tests would confirm your diagnosis?
   (d) Can this condition be treated?

2. This female aged 19 years has several teeth missing.
   (a) What abnormalities do you observe?
   (b) What is the probable cause?
   (c) What further clinical examination would you wish to carry out?
   (d) What further X-ray examination should be made?
   (e) What treatment might be necessary?

Answers on page 73-74

PLATE 19

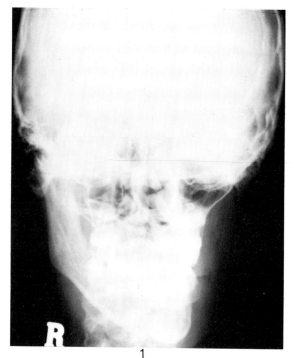

1

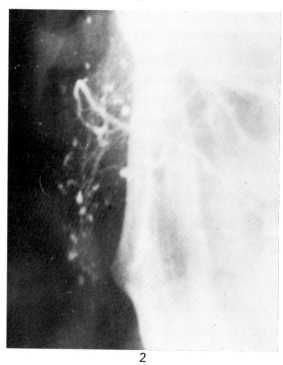

2

PLATE 19

1. **(a)** What is the asymmetrical malformation shown in this antero-posterior view of the mandible? Has it a known family history?
   (b) Is it responsive to early reconstructive surgery?
   (c) Is the incidence 1:1000, 1:4000, 1:8000 live births?

2. This antero-posterior sialogram was carried out on a female patient who complained of dryness of the mouth.
   (a) Which gland is being examined?
   (b) What abnormality is shown?
   (c) What conditions could produce this appearance?
   (d) When is sialography contraindicated?

Answers on page 74

PLATE 20

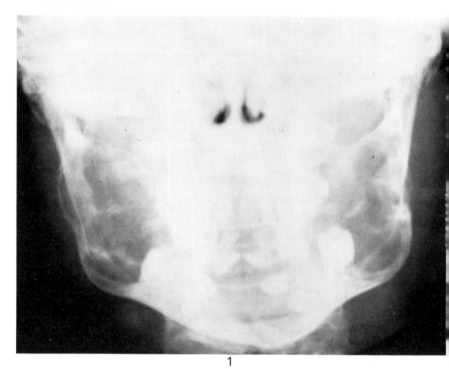

1

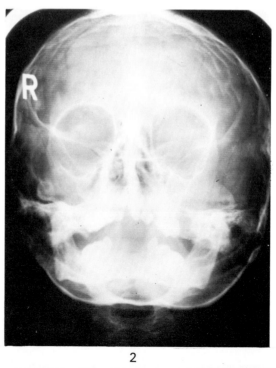

2

PLATE 20

1. **(a)** What abnormality is demonstrated in this antero-posterior view?
   (b) What is the probable diagnosis?
   (c) Could this condition be inherited?
   (d) What changes can be demonstrated in the blood?
   (e) What are the characteristic histological appearances?
   (f) What is the prognosis?

2. The dental abnormalities observed in this radiograph are found in association with frontal bossing, a depressed nasal bridge, prominent ears, thin hair and pouting lips.
   (a) What is this condition, and its cause?
   (b) What additional features may help to distinguish it from congenital syphilis?

Answers on page 74

PLATE 21

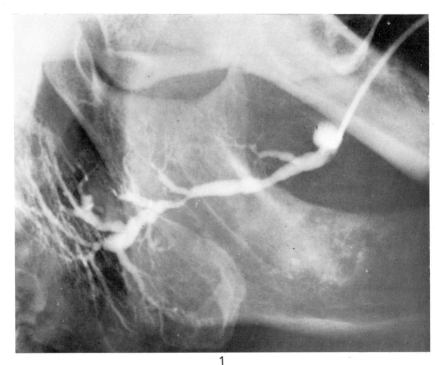

1

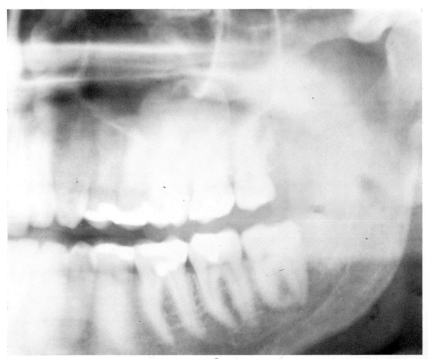

2

PLATE 21

1. **(a)** What is this type of radiographic examination called?
   (b) By what means are radiolucent structures rendered radiopaque?
   (c) What abnormality is demonstrated?
   (d) What could be the cause of the abnormal appearance?

2. This orthopantomograph was requested after an intraoral X-ray revealed a suspected cyst related to the roots of the first and second maxillary molars.
   (a) Describe the abnormality observed in the maxillary sinus.
   (b) Is it rare or common?
   (c) Are the molar teeth vital?
   (d) What treatment is required?

Answers on page 75

PLATE 22

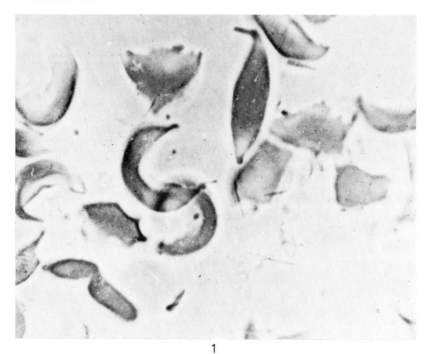

1

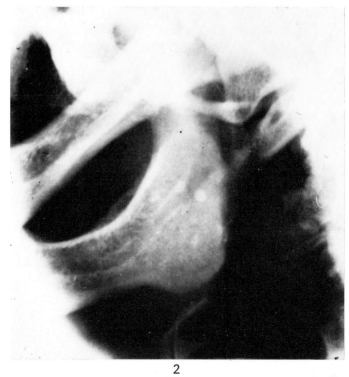

2

PLATE 22

1. This is a blood film showing abnormal red cells.
   (a) What is the abnormality?
   (b) What is this condition called?
   (c) In what racial group is this condition especially prevalent?
   (d) What is the importance of this condition in dental practice?
   (e) What test should be done to identify this condition?

2. **(a)** What abnormality is demonstrated in this lateral oblique radiograph of the mandible?
   (b) Is this likely to be a consequence of **(i)** excess of vitamin D in the diet **(ii)** inhalation of foreign bodies **(iii)** tonsillitis **(iv)** a bee sting **(v)** faulty processing of the X-ray film?

Answers on page 75

PLATE 23

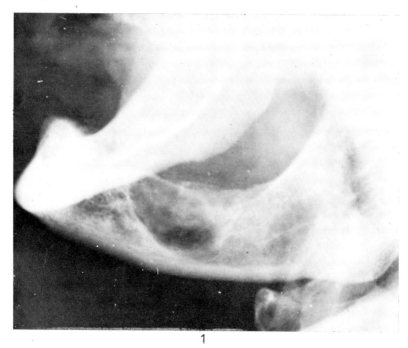

1

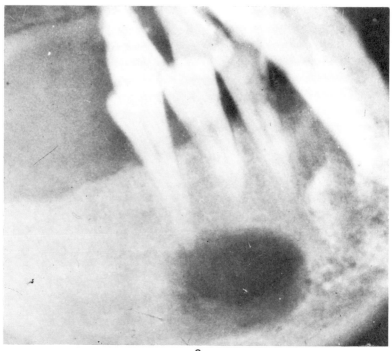

2

PLATE 23

1. This was a lateral view of the mandible in a patient with a history of renal calculi.
   (a) What abnormality is shown?
   (b) What is the probable underlying cause?
   (c) How would you investigate further?
   (d) Can this condition be treated?

2. Radiograph of the jaw of a 60-year-old man who has recently suffered from pleurisy and Cushing's syndrome.
   (a) What abnormality is shown here?
   (b) What condition should be suspected?
   (c) How should the patient be investigated?

Answers on page 76

PLATE 24

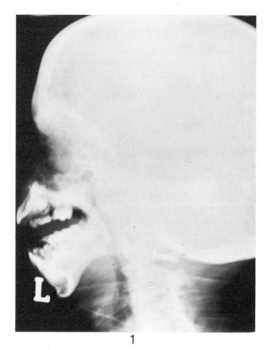

1

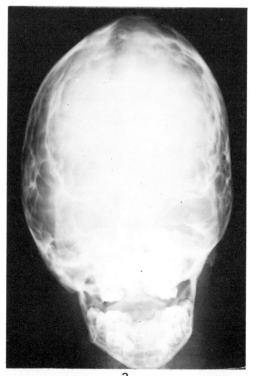

2

PLATE 24

1. This open bite in a bright and intelligent child of eight years has worsened progressively. There is no history of thumb sucking or a persistent tongue thrust.

   (a) In what craniofacial syndrome is this characteristic curvature of the mandible found? Is the condition heritable?

   (b) What other radiological features are characteristic of this condition?

2. (a) What name is given to the unusual bony appearance seen in the skull and in what syndromes is it common?

   (b) Which of the following problems are frequently encountered in such cases: (i) deafness (ii) blindness (iii) prognathism (iv) mental deficiency (v) speech disorders?

Answers on page 76

ANSWER SECTION

PLATE 1

1. (a) Lichen planus. **(b)** Examination of flexor surfaces of skin, forearms and legs. Examination of toe and finger nails. **(c)** Biopsy may be helpful. The typical appearances looked for but found in only about 30-50% of cases are **(i)** hydropic degeneration of basal epithelial cells; **(ii)** proliferation and expansion of prickle cell layer (acanthosis) together with saw-tooth appearance of rete processes; **(iii)** sharply demarcated infiltration of chronic inflammatory cells in the connective tissue directly beneath the basal layers of epithelium; **(iv)** parakeratotic surface.

2. (a) Less severe. **(b)** There is a familial tendency. **(c)** Antibiotics can only alleviate superimposed infection; they do not cure the condition. **(d)** Unlikely. **(e)** Benign migratory glossitis, often referred to as geographical tongue because of its irregular outline.

3. (a) Erosion resulting from rupture of bulla. **(b)** Pemphigoid or pemphigus. **(c)** Biopsy of intact bulla (if present) to demonstrate acantholysis and to see if lesion is intraepithelial (as in pemphigus) or subepithelial (as in benign mucous membrane pemphigoid). Also an immunofluorescent test in pemphigus will demonstrate autoantibodies to intercellular processes of prickle cells whereas in benign mucous membrane pemphigoid autoantibodies, if present, will react with basement membrane. **(d)** This patient had benign mucous membrane pemphigoid with eye lesions but no skin lesions. He responded to treatment with a course of prednisolone starting with a high daily dose and then gradually reducing to a maintenance dose.

4. (a) Severe chronic periodontitis. There is much dental plaque and calculus. There is also a blue-black line on the gingival margin. **(b)** Heavy metal poisoning due to bismuth, lead or mercury. **(c)** Weakness, chronic constipation, anaemia, convulsions and coma. **(d)** All except the fisherman, who is a red herring. Dentists and dental nurses are at risk unless they take appropriate precautions in handling mercury. Miners, welders and smelters are at risk from prolonged inhalation of dust and/or fumes; this patient was an oxyacetylene welder. The connection with prostitution is that heavy metals used to be administered for the treatment of syphilis; with the advent of antibiotics heavy metal poisoning is at least one hazard from which the oldest profession has been freed. It is worth remembering that very young children can also be affected as a result of chewing toys coloured with lead-containing paint.

5. (a) Small inflamed white patch. (b) Combination of white patch with this erythematous base plus bilateral facial rash would suggest chronic discoid lupus erythematosus. (c) Biopsy of white patch may show (i) patchy lymphocytic infiltration and keratosis which may have a pseudo-epitheliomatous appearance (ii) stain with P.A.S. may show characteristic thickening of basement membrane. (d) Treatment of general condition in which steroids and antimalarials are the treatments of choice. Topical steroid such as Triamcinolone acetonide 0.1% in emollient (Adcortyl A in Orabase) for oral lesions.

6. (a) Melanocytes. (b) Neural crest. (c) No, merely more active in the production of melanin. (d) Racial characteristic.

PLATE 2

1. (a) The presence of prominent spider naevi on the skin of the nose and cheeks may be a manifestation of liver failure. (b) (i) Defect in clotting mechanism — prolonged prothrombin time; (ii) risk of spread of serum hepatitis if cirrhosis is secondary to serum hepatitis and patient is a carrier; (iii) any drugs used may not be detoxicated in the liver. (c) The first is impossible; the remainder are highly likely, with alcoholism the primary possibility. The cause of ascites in cirrhosis of the liver is problematical. Anaemia is attributable to blood loss as well as to concomitant hypersplenism.

2. (a) Jaundice. (b) A yellow discolouration of the skin, conjunctivae and mucosa caused by excessive circulating bilirubin, which is a breakdown product of haemoglobin. (c) (i) Haemolytic. (ii) Hepatocellular. (iii) Obstructive. (d) (i) Deficiency of clotting factors causes prolonged prothrombin time; (ii) risk of spread if jaundice is due to serum hepatitis. (iii) Altered response to drugs can occur.

3. **(a)** Leukaemia. **(b)** The tongue is swollen because of the presence of leukaemic infiltration. As a consequence overlying epithelium breaks down and ulcerates. In leukaemia there is decreased resistance to infection. **(c)** The gingivae are swollen because of accumulation of leukaemic cells and inflammation. Bleeding may be related to tissue destruction and also to thrombocytopenia arising as a result of the primitive white cells crowding out the platelet-forming cells in the bone marrow. **(d)** Prevention and control of oral infections by oral hygiene regimes, chlorhexidine mouthwashes, and antifungal agents as required. Dental treatment should be restricted to quiescent periods. When folic acid antagonist drugs such as methotrexate are used, folic acid given topically in the form of folinic acid may help to prevent oral ulceration.

4. **(a)** Stomatitis nicotina. **(b)** The openings of salivary gland ducts are occluded by keratin. **(c)** In general, no. Carcinoma of the palate is rare except in people who practise reverse smoking. **(d)** Abstain from smoking, when the lesions will normally regress.

5. **(a)** Oral mucosa neuroma/thyroid medullary carcinoma syndrome. **(b)** Biopsy of an oral nodule to confirm that the oral lesions are neuromas. Examination of thyroid and tests of thyroid function may be helpful, but the most reliable test is to measure the serum calcitonin. The 'C' cells of the thyroid secrete the hormone. **(c)** Early diagnosis and surgical treatment of the medullary carcinoma is essential and will improve the prognosis for survival. **(d)** Phaeochromocytoma.

6. **(a)** This is the characteristic appearance of hypohidrotic ectodermal dysplasia in which severe hypodontia or anodontia occurs with retarded eruption of the few teeth that may be present. The alveolus does not develop in the absence of teeth and the oral mucosa is dry. **(b)** This syndrome is usually transmitted by females and manifest in males (X-linked recessive). **(c)** Sparse hair, eyebrows and eyelashes; protruberant ears and lips; underdeveloped bridge of nose.

PLATE 3

1. **(a)** Accessory auricles, which are commonly found in many variants of the anomalad now known as hemifacial microsomia. **(b)** All the names listed have been employed to describe the same craniofacial malformation.

2. **(a)** The presence of malar flushing is sometimes indicative of cardiovascular disease especially rheumatic heart disease affecting the mitral valve. It is an indication of incipient cardiac failure and is related to poor venous return. **(b)** Such a patient would be a poor risk for dental surgical operations. The pationt should probably be hospitalised and general anaesthesia in such cases calls for particular care.

3. **(a)** Decreased salivary gland function or dietary factors are two obvious possibilities to account for rampant caries. In this case it was decreased salivary gland function due to Sjogren syndrome. Cervical caries and gross tooth destruction are typical of changes seen in severe xerostomia; this, together with changes in salivary composition, may account for gross caries in uncontrolled diabetics. Investigations should include **(i)** salivary — such tests of salivary function as flow rate, labial biopsy and sialography; **(ii)** dietary — investigations of dietary history by careful questioning and requiring the patient to fill in diet sheets. **(b)** **(i)** Preventive dental treatment — plaque control methods and topical fluoride applications; **(ii)** dietary advice and supervision; **(iii)** regular dental treatment at three-monthly intervals or less.

4. **(a)** Membranous glossitis with candida infection. Brown discolouration is present in crusts on the tongue surface. **(b)** Bad or metallic taste and characteristic odour, both related to the high concentration of urea in the mouth and its breakdown to ammonia. These patients are prone to infections — bacterial and fungal. Petechiae of the palate and bleeding from the gingivae are possibly related to thrombocytopenia but other haemostatic factors are also abnormal. **(c)** Uncertain, but apart from infections probably not common. **(d)** The oral condition will be improved by treating the cause of the renal failure and uraemia. If this is irreversible, dialysis or renal transplantation may be required. Oral infections should be anticipated and prevented or treated where they occur.

5. **(a)** Acromegaly; due to excessive output of growth hormone by an eosinophil cell tumour of the anterior pituitary occurring after the skeletal epiphyses have fused. **(b)** Enlargement of tongue, hands, feet, head and supra-orbital ridges. **(c)** Diabetes and hypertension. **(d)** Skull radiographs show prominent frontal ridges, enlarged air sinuses and pituitary fossa (which may also show erosion of clinoid processes). **(e)** Where progressive and when complications are difficult to control, destruction of the tumour is effected by surgical resection, implant of a radioisotope, cryosurgery or irradiation.

6. **(a)** Actinomycosis. **(b)** *Actinomyces israelii.* **(c)** By examination of pus from the abscesses. Sulphur-like granules may be seen on macroscopic examination of the pus; smears show Gram positive branching filaments sometimes with terminal clubs. Organisms can be cultured anaerobically. **(d)** Lungs, caecum, liver. **(e)** **(i)** Abscesses require incision and drainage; **(ii)** penicillin or tetracycline in high dosage and for periods of 1-2 months, or longer where bone is infected.

PLATE 4

1. **(a)** The puffiness of the face, especially the periorbital areas, is typical of myxoedema, or hypothyroidism. **(b)** It is due to the accumulation of mucins in the subcutaneous tissues. It does not pit on pressure. **(c)** Patients with myxoedema often have ischaemic heart disease associated with high serum cholesterol levels. They may also have respiratory disease. Anaesthesia for dental surgical procedures requires careful consideration.

2. **(a)** Telangiectatic spots on dorsal surface of tongue. **(b)** Hereditary Haemorrhagic Telangiectasia (Osler-Weber-Rendu Disease). **(c)** It is an inherited disorder transmitted as a simple dominant and therefore is usually familial. **(d)** Skin and mucosa of nose, mouth, gastro-intestinal, respiratory and renal tracts. **(e)** If areas are traumatised haemorrhages occur and may lead to iron-deficiency anaemia. **(f)** Yes; repeated cryotherapy to the lesions can be used to prevent problems of bleeding.

3. **(a)** Pink coloured palms which may be associated with advanced liver disease. **(b)** The significance of liver disease in dental practice includes: bleeding tendency due to reduced production of clotting factors with a prolonged prothrombin time; patient may have had serum hepatitis and may be a carrier; altered response to drugs, as many are detoxicated in the liver. Alcoholics may have considerable resistance to anaesthetic agents.

4. (a) Avitaminosis C. **(b)** Scurvy occurred commonly among sailors deprived of fresh food during long voyages. **(c)** Subclinical scurvy can occur in the elderly — again, for lack of fresh food in the diet. **(d)** Paucity of collagen fibres and evidence of capillary fragility.

5. (a) (i) Biopsy. **(ii)** Ascertain whether the patient has an exanthematous fever. This term is given to the appearance of the tongue in the early stages of scarlet fever. It is due to swelling of the fungiform papillae against the background of a coated tongue. **(iii)** Dark ground illumination of a smear. **(iv)** History. **(b)** History would exclude **(ii)** and **(iv)**; followed by examination of a smear; finally, biopsy. In this instance the lesion is a syphilitic chancre.

6. (a) Mild glossitis of tongue tip. **(b)** Hypochromic anaemia. **(c)** Serum iron and total iron binding capacity to determine iron saturation. **(d) (i)** Identify the underlying cause and treat it; **(ii)** oral iron e.g. ferrous sulphate, 200 mg 3x daily; **(iii)** severe cases may need parenteral iron or blood transfusions.

PLATE 5

1. (a) Vesicular eruption on palate. **(b)** Herpes simplex, herpangina, or other viral disease. **(c)** Smears and swabs for viral isolation and an initial blood sample for serological examination to be followed after 14 days by a further blood sample. **(d)** Both herpes and herpangina usually remit within 7-10 days, and treatment is essentially symptomatic — bed rest, soft diet, oral hygiene, mouthwashes. If lesions persist, antiviral agents such as idoxuridine might be used for herpes simplex infections, but their effectiveness is by no means assured.

2. (a) Oral bulla. **(b)** A biopsy while bulla is still intact. Intact bullae give much more diagnostic information than ruptured ones. **(c)** Indirect or direct immunofluorescent techniques to demonstrate autoantibodies to intercellular substance of stratum spinosum (pemphigus vulgaris) or to basement membrane (pemphigoid). With the direct test a sample of patient's mucosa or skin is also required. **(d)** Skin, eyes and vagina.

3. **(a)** Facial paralysis on the right side. **(b)** Bell's palsy. **(c)** Ramsay Hunt Syndrome. Melkersson-Rosenthal Syndrome. **(d)** None; **(iv)** is most popularly offered as an explanation for this sudden and inexplicable affliction.

4. **(a)** Antimongoloid slope of the orbits, notching of the outer third of the lower eyelids, malar hypoplasia, low-set ears and a tongue-shaped extension of hair towards the cheek are all pathognomonic of Treacher Collins syndrome (mandibulofacial dysostosis). **(b)** Severe anterior open bite usually accompanies the marked curvature of the lower border of the mandible found in this familial syndrome.

5. **(a)** The origins of median rhomboid glossitis are uncertain. **(b)** It was thought to represent an abnormal persistence of the tuberculum impar. **(c)** As the lesion often appears only in adult life, and as the site does not always correspond to that of the tuberculum impar, the possibility has been suggested that this is a form of atrophic glossitis associated with candidal infection. **(d)** It is not commonly premalignant.

6. **(a)** Finger clubbing. **(b)** Bronchiectasis and congenital heart diseases. It is usually an indication of suppurative respiratory disease or long-standing cyanotic disease of cardiac origin. **(c)** Dental treatment in such patients requires careful planning and prophylactic antibiotic therapy. Cardiac or respiratory disease limits the availability of general anaesthesia. In addition congenital heart disease exposes the patient to the danger of developing bacterial endocarditis — in the pathogenesis of which oral micro-organisms are frequently implicated. (For an interesting comment on this condition see an editorial in *Brit. Med J.,* Vol. 2, p.785, September 14, 1977).

1. (a) Mucocele. (b) Yes. It may also occur in the buccal mucosa or floor of the mouth. (c) Presence of mucus, of a lumen lined by connective tissue, and of related salivary tissue. (d) Mechanical trauma to ducts of minor salivary glands.

2. (a) Lichen planus, reticular type. (b) Atrophic, bullous, erosive, papular, plaque. (c) 1M:2F.

3. (a) Condylar hypoplasia. Coloboma of the upper lid and epibulbar dermoids indicate that this is a case of Goldenhar syndrome, a variant of hemifacial microsomia. Those who gave other answers could learn much about these rather confusing craniofacial syndromes by consulting *Syndromes of the Head and Neck* by Gorlin, Pindborg and Cohen, McGraw Hill, New York, 1976.

4. (a) Vesicular eruption beneath upper denture on the patient's right side; vesicles have ruptured on the left side. (b) This patient was receiving cytotoxic drug therapy for malignant disease and was therefore immunosuppressed.

5. (a) Chronic hyperplastic gingivitis. (b) Phenytoin sodium (Dilantin, Epanutin). (c) For control of epileptic seizures. (d) Fibrous hyperplasia with superimposed inflammatory changes following food stagnation and plaque. (e) Improved oral hygiene, removal of any local irritation. In established cases surgical excision of hyperplastic gingivae may be necessary. The possibility of drug substitution with e.g. Primidone (mysoline) should be discussed with the patient's medical practitioner and physician.

6. (a) Tuberculosis. Biopsy to demonstrate tubercle follicles with epithelioid cells and Langhans type giant cells. The biopsy can be stained by Ziehl-Neelsen's method to demonstrate the pink acid and alcohol fast tubercle bacilli. Culture on Lowenstein-Jensen's medium and animal inoculation may also be attempted. (b) Lungs should be X-rayed. Sputum should also be examined. (c) Oral lesions are usually secondary to primary lung infections and rapidly clear up when systemic chemotherapy is effective.

PLATE 7

1. (a) Smooth fissured tongue. Some surface debris is also present. **(b)** When patients complain of persistent dryness of the mouth a full case history, including drug history, is required. They should be asked specifically about the other signs or symptoms of Sjogren syndrome; for example any abnormalities of eyes, such as recurrent dry or 'gritty' sensation or eye infections, and also any history of arthritis or joint stiffness. **(c)** This will vary according to the facilities available but ideally would include salivary flow rate measurement, labial gland biopsy, and sialography. **(d)** Serological tests for circulating autoantibodies such as rheumatoid factor and antinuclear factor.

2. (a) Diffuse stomatitis with superficial exudate as seen in erythema multiforme. **(b)** Drug sensitivity e.g. sulphonamides or barbiturates, or viral infection such as herpes simplex. In fact it was a primary herpetic gingivostomatitis in a young adult. **(c)** Viral smear and culture. Primary serum collected followed by convalescent about 14 days later should show a four-fold rise in serum antibody titre.

3. (a) Antibiotic sore tongue due to suppression of normal flora permitting overgrowth of Candida albicans. **(b)** Smear and stain with Gram to show hyphae of Candida albicans. Swab cultured on Sabouraud's medium selectively allows growth of colonies. **(c)** Amphotericin B (10 mg lozenges) 4 x daily until signs and symptoms resolve.

4. (a) Recurrent aphthae. **(b)** In Behcet syndrome eye and genital lesions may occur. **(c)** In chronic more severe cases blood examination including erythrocyte sedimentation rate, haemoglobin, absolute values (mean corpuscular volume, mean corpuscular haemoglobin), film, as well as serum vitamin B12, whole blood folate and iron saturation. **(d)** Various topical applications have been used, for example: Chlorhexidine mouthwash, Zinc sulphate and Zinc chloride mouthwash, Sodium perborate, Hydrocortisone Lozenges, B.P.C. (Corlan Pellets), Triamcinolone Dental Paste, B.P.C. (Adcortyl in Orabase).

5. (a) Leukoplakia or squamous cell carcinoma. **(b)** Speckled appearance is suggestive of malignant tendency. **(c)** Palpation of cervical lymph glands. **(d)** Biopsy.

6. (a) Perforation of palate. **(b)** In this age group the breakdown of a syphilitic gumma is the most likely cause but tuberculosis should also be considered. **(c) (i)** Serological test for syphilis — Complement Fixation Test (Wassermann), Fluorescent Treponemal Antibody Test, Treponema Immobilisation Test; **(ii)** biopsy of the lesion may demonstrate the typical histological features of a syphilitic gumma — necrosis, cellular infiltration of lymphocytes and plasma cells, and periarteritis and endarteritis.

Answers to questions on page 17

PLATE 8

1. **(a)** Myasthenia gravis. (In which choline instead of depolarising the motor end plate as normally happens actually competes with acetylcholine and causes neuromuscular block). **(b)** By the history and by the demonstration of a response to anticholinesterase. **(c)** Yes, with neostigmine, an anticholinesterase drug which allows acetylcholine produced at neuro-muscular end plates to be potentiated. **(d)** Thymectomy provides the best chance of a permanent cure more especially in the younger age groups.

2. **(a)** Ulceration and purpuric areas. **(b)** Could occur in diseases where there is both haemorrhagic tendency and increased susceptibility to infection e.g. marrow aplasia, leukaemia. **(c)** Blood examination including erythrocyte sedimentation rate, haemoglobin, absolute values (M.C.V., M.C.H.), film, differential white count, platelet count. Bone marrow examination will be necessary. **(d)** Swollen and bleeding gums, ulceration and infection. In this instance herpes virus was isolated from the labial lesions.

3. **(a)** Von Recklinghausen's neurofibromatosis. **(b)** *Cafe au lait* pigmentation of the trunk. **(c)** Yes, and frequently do. **(d)** Malignant transformation of neurofibromata may occur, especially those involving deeper structures, but sarcomatous change is less common in the oral region.

4. **(a)** Sialosis. **(b) (i)** Liver cirrhosis especially alcoholic cirrhosis; **(ii)** malnutrition, especially protein deficiency; **(iii)** drug induced e.g. some adrenaline-like drugs, such as isoprenaline used in treatment of bronchial asthma and bronchospasm; **(iv)** endocrine, e.g. diabetes mellitus as in this case where it was the

first manifestation of disease. **(c)** Varies according to the cause and whether it can be eliminated. In this case it was relieved by treatment of diabetes mellitus. (For further reading on sialosis consult *Salivary Glands in Health and Disease* by D. K. Mason and D. M. Chisholm. W. B. Saunders Co. Ltd., 1975).

5. **(a)** Circular iris-like lesions of erythema multiforme. **(b)** Extensive inflammation of lips and mucosa with patchy ulceration. **(c)** Uncertain: drug hypersensitivity and viral infection e.g. herpes simplex have been suggested. **(d)** If an infective cause can be excluded by virological tests then local or systemic steroids may be of value.

6. **(a)** Rheumatoid arthritis. **(b)** Dryness of the mouth, salivary gland swelling and pain or stiffness of the temporomandibular joint. **(c)** Some patients may be or may have been on prolonged steroid therapy so that the normal increase in endogenous steroid output does not occur in response to the stress of general anaesthesia and dental surgical procedures. Some hypotension may occur unless the steroid dosage is increased. Furthermore, rheumatoid involvement of the cervical spine often occurs and forceful extension of the neck during general anaesthesia can have serious consequences.

PLATE 9

1. **(a)** Florid complexion with some cyanosis and red conjunctivae suggest polycythaemia. **(b)** An abnormal increase in the number of red cells may occur spontaneously in a primary form, or secondarily to compensate for the effects of chronic tissue anoxia, e.g. in chronic bronchitis, emphysema, congenital heart disease, at high altitude. **(c)** Sluggish blood flow, hypertension, cerebral thrombosis. **(d)** Significant bleeding may follow dental extraction.

2. **(a)** Ramsay Hunt Syndrome. **(b)** *Herpes zoster* affecting facial nerve (geniculate ganglion). **(c)** Shingles refers to *herpes zoster* infection of sensory nerves. **(d)** Taste, in about 50% of cases. **(e)** Symptomatic only. The vesicles should be kept dry and free from infection. Analgesics can be administered for relief of pain. Prognosis is good; complete recovery is usual within several weeks, but can be delayed for up to two years.

3. **(a)** Fordyce spots. **(b)** Developmental abnormality. These are ectopic sebaceous glands. **(c)** Buccal mucosa. **(d)** None, apart from reassuring the patient.

4. **(a)** Peutz-Jeghers syndrome. **(b)** Intestinal polyposis. **(c)** All are related to the polyposis — bleeding, intestinal obstruction, intussusception, malignant transformation of polyps. **(d)** Periorbitally, perinasally, hands and feet.

5. **(a)** Blue sclerae. **(b)** Because of defective formation of connective tissue matrix the sclerae are abnormally thin and allow the underlying pigmented tissue to shine through. **(c)** Dentinogenesis imperfecta. **(d)** No, the patient can only be protected as much as possible from further fractures.

6. **(a)** In this age group a haemangioma is most probable but a mucocele or a salivary tumour is also possible. This was a cavernous haemangioma. **(b)** Pressure on the lesion may cause it to blanch as the venous blood is pressed out. **(c)** Surgical removal or cryosurgery (which obviates the risk of excessive blood loss).

PLATE 10

1. **(a)** Sarcoidosis. **(b)** Increased erythrocyte sedimentation rate would be expected. Also leucopenia, eosinophilia, thrombocytopenia, hyperproteinaemia and hypercalcaemia may occur. The elevated serum proteins are due to elevated alpha-2, beta and gamma globulins. **(c)** There is a deficiency in the delayed type cutaneous sensitivity. To assist in reaching a diagnosis two skin tests are useful: **(i)** Kveim Test — performed by the intradermal injection of 0.2ml Kveim antigen in the forearm. After 6 weeks the site (which has to be accurately marked) is excised and the typical sarcoid granuloma signifies a positive reaction; **(ii)** Mantoux Test — the majority of patients with sarcoid are negative tuberculin reactors. **(d)** Subacute sarcoidosis will often resolve spontaneously but the chronic form of the disease is a much more serious problem. Treatment with corticosteroids will suppress the effects of the disease but requires to be continued over a period of years. Oral lesions require careful hygiene until the systemic therapy takes effect.

2. **(a)** Erythema multiforme. **(b)** Cause is unknown. Certain drugs (e.g. sulphonamides and barbiturates) have been

incriminated. A viral aetiology has also been suggested. **(c)** Fever, constitutional disturbance; skin, eyes, and genitalia may also be affected. **(d)** Steroids topically or systemically. An episode usually lasts about three weeks. **(e)** Yes, about one in three cases recurs.

3. **(a)** Squamous carcinoma, leukoplakia and lichen planus. **(b)** Biopsy examination is essential. **(c)** The discoid form of lupus erythematosus may mimic the appearance of this candidal leukoplakia. Leukoplakia was formerly considered to be particularly common in syphilitics but it may well be that this was a result of treatment (with heavy metals) rather than an association with the disease process. Options **(i)**, **(ii)** and **(iv)** deserve to be dismissed with scorn.

4. **(a)** Beefy tongue or glossitis. **(b)** Deficiency of vitamin B12 or folic acid. **(c) (i)** Further blood examination — whole blood folate and serum B12; **(ii)** if serum B12 is low then bone marrow examination and Schilling tests will be required, as well as augmented histamine test of gastric function; **(iii)** tests for malabsorption may be indicated. **(d)** Sub-acute combined degeneration of the spinal cord and peripheral neuritis.

5. **(a)** These are foliate papillae. They contain lymphoid tissue. Some of the papillae are slightly inflamed and this could be termed foliate papillitis, probably due to trauma or food stagnation. **(b)** Hot saline mouthwashes 4 x daily to reduce inflammation. **(c)** Cancerophobia — and not without some justification since this is a relatively common site of oral cancer.

6. **(a)** A manifestation of oral candida infection following immunosuppression induced by cytotoxic drugs. **(b)** If patches are easily rubbed off a smear stained with Gram could demonstrate Gram positive hyphae of Candida albicans. If patches are thickened and adherent, a biopsy stained with P.A.S. could demonstrate hyphae in superficial layers of epithelium. **(c)** The denture should be left out as much as possible. A course of Amphotericin B (10 mg lozenges) sucked 4 x daily should be prescribed until the infection clears. Amphotericin B cream can be applied to the fitting surface of the denture when it is being worn.

1. (a) Recurrent aphthae — minor type. **(b)** Fordyce spots. **(c) (i)** Exclude menstrually related aphthae by history. **(ii)** Exclude nutritional deficiency by blood examinations: Haemoglobin, absolute values (mean corpuscular volume, mean corpuscular haemoglobin), film, erythrocyte sedimentation rate, serum vitamin B12, whole blood folate, serum iron and total iron binding capacity for iron saturation. **(d)** Use chlorhexidine mouthwash *or* zinc sulphate mouthwash B.P.C., *or* topical steroids, for example: Corlan pellets, Adcortyl in Orabase.

2. (a) Small flat polygonal papules, reddish-violet to brown, and glistening. **(b)** Lichen planus. **(c)** White patches often with a reticular pattern (see Plate 1 fig. 1, Plate 6 fig. 2) characteristically affecting the buccal and labial mucosa, but the tongue and gingivae may also be involved. About 20% of cases are of the atrophic or erosive type. Bullous types may also occur, but infrequently. **(d)** Toe and finger nails; hair follicle involvement may cause baldness. **(e)** No; the figures reported are very variable but skin lesions are probably present in less than half the cases with oral lesions.

3. (a) Cheilitis granulomatosa. **(b)** Uncertain. Excluding the possibility of local trauma, it may be part of Melkersson-Rosenthal Syndrome where either fissuring of the tongue or facial palsy may also occur. It can occur in sarcoidosis. It may be an early oral or facial manifestation of Crohn's disease (see Carr, D., [1974] *Brit Med J,* 4: 636). In this instance the diagnosis proved to be Crohn's disease. **(c)** Intra-lesional or systemic steroids have been helpful in some cases.

4. (a) Hemifacial microsomia. **(b)** It arises early in the first trimester of pregnancy. The congenital malformation of the left ear in association with mandibular hypoplasia and maxillary under-development distinguished this condition from birth forceps trauma, postnatal infection of the mandibular condyle or juvenile ostomyelitis of the mandible. **(c)** One birth in 3500. **(d)** Disordered development of the first and second branchial arches due to a vascular accident in the vicinity of the stapedial arterial stem; it is not familial. **(e)** Reconstruction with costo-chondral grafts — after growth is complete on the normal side.

5. (a) Recurrent candidiasis. Confirmation could be sought from a smear and a culture. **(b)** Recurrence of *Candida albicans* infection suggests that either a local or a systemic underlying cause persists. It is, therefore, essential to reconsider such a patient's history and to carry out a careful clinical examination. It is important to consider drug history, endocrine status, malnutrition, malabsorption, haematological deficiency; also to examine for any other possible manifestations such as involvement of skin, nails and vagina. **(c)** Full blood examination including erythrocyte sedimentation rate, haemoglobin, absolute values, film, and iron saturation. Tests of cellular and humoral immune mechanisms should also be considered as an immune defect, congenital or acquired, may be implicated.

6. **(a)** Angular cheilitis. **(b)** Ill-fitting dentures with loss of vertical dimension. It may be associated with stomatitis. **(c)** *Candida albicans* or *Staphylococcus aureus.* See MacFarlane & Helnarska [1976] *Brit Dent J,* 140, 403). **(d)** Avitaminosis; cheilitis is seen particularly in riboflavin deficiency. Readers guessing oligiasis have been trapped; there is no such disease. Those opting for measles may be thinking of Koplik's spots, which occur intraorally. The white scaly patches of psoriasis are usually symmetrical, and very rarely affect the oral mucosa.

PLATE 12

1. **(a)** Swelling in the submandibular region suggests that the patient has developed lymphoma. **(b)** About 5-10%. **(c)** The diagnosis of lymphoma can be difficult, but the following points should be considered in making a diagnosis: **(i)** Sjogren syndrome patients most liable to develop lymphoma appear to be those with the sicca complex, i.e. dry eyes and dry mouth only, with high levels of circulating autoantibodies and who have had radiotherapy for salivary gland enlargement; **(ii)** in some cases the onset of lymphoma coincides with marked reduction in levels of circulating autoantibodies, such as rheumatoid and antinuclear factor, which commonly occur in Sjogren syndrome; **(iii)** biopsy of the swelling. The early appearances in lymphomatous change have been described (Azzopardi, J. C. and Evans, D. J. [1971], *J Clin Path,* 24: 744) and include the presence of histiocytes and foci of necrosis, as well as immature lymphocytes.

2. **(a)** Sialorrhoea (ptyalism). (Note accumulation of salivary froth on the palate). **(b)** Much less common than xerostomia. **(c)** Tooth eruption; ulcerative stomatitis. **(d)** Heavy metal poisoning; epilepsy; Parkinsonism; schizophrenia. Drooling may however be a reflection of impaired muscle control rather than excessive secretion of saliva.

3. **(a)** All except condylar aplasia and bifid tongue may be found in Crouzon syndrome (craniofacial dysostosis) where incomplete development of cranial sutures produces severe maxillary hypoplasia and secondary dental defects. **(b)** Blindness, from optic nerve involvement in severe cases of exophthalmos, is the major threat and is relieved by craniofacial surgery.

4. **(a)** *Candida albicans.* The hyphae are characteristic of the pathogenic form of the fungus. They are Gram positive. **(b)** Yes. Sabouraud's medium, which has a low pH and inhibits the growth of many common oral bacteria. **(c)** Denture sore mouth, angular cheilitis, thrush, antibiotic stomatitis, candidal leukoplakia. **(d)** Antifungal agents such as Nystatin or Amphotericin B. **(e)** Antibiotics, steroids, cytotoxic drugs, and possibly drugs which promote dry mouth as an undesirable side effect.

5. **(a)** Albright syndrome. Swelling of maxilla may be only one of several bony sites showing features of fibrous dysplasia. **(b)** Endocrine dysfunction, precocious sexual development, and areas of pigmentation of the skin similar to that illustrated.

6. **(a)** Pigmented areas and the history of general lassitude suggest the possibility of Addison's disease. **(b)** Pigmented patches of skin — especially areas of skin folds, sites exposed to friction (e.g. belt areas), and normally pigmented sites (e.g. nipples, axillae). **(c)** Melanin. **(d)** Ascertain whether there are low plasma cortisol levels and a lack of adrenal cortical response to adrenocorticotrophic hormone (A.C.T.H.). Low urinary output and greatly diminished urinary steroids are strongly suggestive of Addison's disease.

PLATE 13

1. **(a)** Traumatic. Related to sharp edge of a carious molar tooth. **(b)** Parotid duct orifice. **(c)** Removal of cause, viz. filling the carious tooth.

2. **(a)** Fibrous dysplasia. **(b)** X-ray and biopsy. **(c)** Conservatively, as it tends to stop growing when the child does. Bone paring for aesthetic reasons is usually all that is required after body growth has ceased. **(d)** Albright syndrome — polyostotic fibrous dysplasia — skin pigmentation — precocious puberty.

3. **(a)** Exophthalmos. **(b)** Thyrotoxicosis. **(c)** Hazards associated with cardiac failure, atrial fibrillation and extreme anxiety. Surgical treatment and stress should be avoided until thyrotoxicosis is controlled by such measures as drug therapy, surgery or radioiodine treatment.

4. **(a)** Mumps or epidemic parotitis. **(b)** Mumps virus. **(c)** Droplet infection. **(d)** Complement fixation will identify virus in saliva and serum during the first week. **(e)** Pancreatitis, orchitis, oophoritis, meningitis.

5. **(a)** Numerous large immature white blood cells. The cell in the centre is undergoing mitosis. **(b)** Acute or chronic leukaemia. Monocytic, myeloid, lymphocytic leukaemia. **(c)** Swellings, ulceration, bleeding, infection. **(d)** Uncertain: according to reports 15-85% of patients with leukaemia have oral manifestations; spontaneous gingival haemorrhage can be the first symptom of the disease, especially in its acute form.

6. **(a)** Anaemia, hypertension, widespread vascular disease due to atheroma. They may have acquired defects of cellular immunity and are prone to infections. Also they have increased risk of exposure to serum hepatitis. **(b) (i)** If they are exposed to the virus of serum hepatitis they may become long term carriers. It is important in dental treatment to prevent cross infection via saliva, blood or infective materials. Adequate precautions would include protection of the patient by the cleaning and sterilising of instruments and disposal of waste materials, and also protection of the clinician by using disposable gowns, gloves, mask and glasses. (For further information see *Cross Infection and Sterilisation in General Practice,* MacFarlane, T. W. *Brit Dent. J.,* 1976, 141; 213.)

1. (a) (i) Iron saturation is low — values under 16% are
subnormal; (ii) whole blood folate is low — levels below 80 ug/l
are abnormally low; (iii) serum vitamin B12 is normal — values
under 120 ng/l are abnormally low. (b) Adult
coeliac disease — a form of malabsorption associated with
gluten hypersensitivity. (c) This patient should be referred to
a physician for further investigation of gastrointestinal
function (xylose and fat absorption, intestinal biopsy) and
bone marrow function. (d) Iron and folate supplements and a
gluten free diet. (For further information see Wray *et al. Brit Med
J* 1975, 1: 490.)

2. (a) Ring staining of erythrocytes; some target cells are also
present. (b) Glossitis and angular cheilitis; candida infection
and oral ulceration have also been reported. (c) Plummer-
Vinson or Kelly-Paterson syndrome. (d) Determine
haemoglobin level, mean corpuscular volume, mean
corpuscular haemoglobin, serum iron, total iron binding
capacity for iron saturation. If dysphagia is present a barium
swallow X-ray and oesophagoscopy is necessary to exclude
post-cricoid carcinoma, a complication of Plummer-Vinson
syndrome.

3. (a) Skin bullae. (b) Pemphigus, bullous pemphigoid or benign
mucous membrane pemphigoid. If skin only is involved
bullous pemphigoid is the most likely diagnosis. (c) Biopsy of a
skin bulla to ascertain whether it was intra-epithelial
(pemphigus) or sub-epithelial (pemphigoid). Fluorescent
antibody test could also be helpful. (d) Internal malignancy.

4. (a) Hodgkin's disease. (b) Enlargement of spleen and lymph
nodes in other parts of the body. (c) Chest X-ray to see if
mediastinal lymph nodes are enlarged. (d) Biopsy of an
enlarged cervical lymph node to reveal typical cellular
changes including presence of characteristic giant cells. (e)
Variable and uncertain prognosis. Survival varies from
months to 20-30 years after appropriate radiotherapy.

5. (a) Vesicular eruption. (b) Herpes simplex gingivostomatitis.
(c) Not usually the oral mucosa; recurrent form affects lips —
herpes labialis. (d) (i) A stained smear from a recent vesicle
shows degenerating nuclei containing inclusion bodies
clustered together to form swollen giant cells. (ii) Virus
isolation. Virus can be grown in tissue culture. (iii)
Serologically by demonstrating a greater than four-fold rise

in titre after 14-21 days. **(e)** Mainly symptomatic. The patient should be reassured, and advised to adopt a soft diet. If constitutionally upset the patient should be kept in bed. Tetracycline mouthwashes 250 mgm. 4 x daily for adults, quarter dose for children, is said to give symptomatic relief.

6. **(a)** Acute ulcerative gingivitis of the Vincent's type. The clinical appearance of the interdental papillae is typical and there is a characteristic fetor oris. **(b)** Smears show Vincent's organisms — spirochaetes and fusiform bacilli — in profusion in most cases. A positive smear is only diagnostic in conjunction with the clinical appearance. (Note. Smears are best treated by the simplest staining method — staining with dilute carbol fuchsin. There is no point in taking a swab as the organisms are extremely difficult to culture.)

PLATE 15

1. **(a)** Macroglossia. **(b)** Amyloid deposition is a complication of myelomatosis and may cause macroglossia. **(c)** Stains to disclose the presence of amyloid (e.g. Congo Red, which produces green birefringence when viewed under polarized light; thioflavine T, which produces fluorescence under ultraviolet light; methyl violet, which may produce a metachromatic appearance). **(d)** Presence of abnormal serum and urinary proteins. Presence of abnormal plasma cells in bone marrow. Presence of punched out osteolytic areas in skeleton, especially skull, ribs and vertebrae.

2. **(a)** Lichen planus. **(b)** Skin, especially flexor surfaces of forearms and legs. Finger and toe nails. **(c)** Stress has been suggested as an aetiological factor and this should be eliminated where possible. Oral lesions in the chronic form of the condition, as in this case, tend to persist with or without steroid treatment for months to years. The skin lesions respond well to topical steroid therapy.

3. **(a)** Koilonychia or spooning of the finger nails. **(b)** Iron deficiency anaemia. **(c)** F > M. **(d)** Glossitis and dysphagia. This may progress to oesophageal stricture and post-cricoid carcinoma. Plummer-Vinson or Kelly-Patterson syndrome.

4. **(a)** Herpes labialis. **(b)** *Herpes simplex* virus. **(c)** Between attacks the virus is believed to reside in the trigeminal ganglion and nerve tissue. **(d)** Trauma, sunlight, respiratory

disease, other systemic illness, immunosuppressed states.
(e) Frequent topical administration of anaesthetic ether at the
first symptom of a developing herpetic lesion has been found
helpful in some cases. (See Sabin, A.B. Misery of recurrent
herpes: what to do? *New Engl. J. Med.* 293: 986-988 Nov. 6,
1975.)

5. (a) Corticosteroids. (b) Rheumatoid arthritis and other
connective tissue disease, bronchial asthma, and in many
other conditions where the immunosuppressive effect is
helpful. (c) Adrenal suppression could occur and the
necessary increase in secretion during dental surgical
treatment or during dental anaesthesia would not be
forthcoming. Hypotension and death could ensue. (d) By
giving steroid before and, if necessary, during the operation.

6. (a) Dehydration, decreased salivary gland function or, rarely,
calculus in the duct. (b) Staphylococcus and streptococcus
pyogenes. (c) (i) Obtain a specimen of pus for bacteriology;
blood cultures if systemic effects are in evidence. (ii) Early
therapy with cloxacillin, as penicillin-resistant organisms are
likely to be involved. If Gram negative septicaemia is
suspected, a broad spectrum antibiotic such as cephalothin
should be given. This can be altered when results of
antibiotic sensitivity are obtained. (iii) Supportive therapy —
rehydration, oral hygiene, analgesics and avoidance of drugs
which might reduce salivary flow. (iv) Surgical drainage may
be required. (d) Sialography.

Answers to questions on page 33

PLATE 16

1. (a) Menstrually related recurrent aphthae. (b) About a week
before menstruation. (c) Few days to a week after
menstruation. (d) The use of synthetic hormone preparations.
These should only be prescribed after the individual patient's
case has been fully discussed with the patient's general
medical practitioner and a gynaecologist. The morbidity of the
ulcers, the obstetric history and aspirations of the patient, as
well as gynaecological history have all to be considered.

2. (a) Smear and swab for microbiological examination. This is
an acute candida infection. The smear may be stained with
Gram; the swab is plated out on Sabouraud's medium. (b)
Amphotericin B lozenges (10 mg) sucked 4 x daily after meals
for three weeks and Amphotericin B cream applied to
affected areas of lips and denture-bearing surfaces. (c)
Variable. These severe cases may recur and underlying
causes of oral candidiasis should be sought such as drug

induced, acquired immune defects, endocrine disease, as well as local factors such as ill-fitting dentures. The possibility of malignant change (as in this case) in the affected oral mucosa should be borne in mind.

3. **(a)** Systemic or discoid lupus erythematosus. **(b) (i)** Dryness of the mouth; **(ii)** inflamed areas with a tendency to ulcerate; **(iii)** inflamed areas speckled with adherent white reticular patches. **(c)** Biopsy.

4. **(a) (i)** Benign mucous membrane pemphigoid (oral bullae); **(ii)** Behcet syndrome (oral ulceration); **(iii)** Sjogren syndrome (dry mouth, oral candidiasis and salivary swelling); **(iv)** Stevens-Johnson syndrome (extensive oral erythema, erosions, ulcerations).

5. **(a)** Squamous carcinoma. Any ulcerating lesion that has not healed after so long a period, even were it not enlarging, should be regarded as malignant until proved otherwise. **(b)** The ulcer is indurated and fixed to underlying and adjacent tissues; enlarged local lymph nodes would be a further sign. **(c)** Radiotherapy and chemotherapy. (For recent advances in these fields see the paper on use of fast neutrons by Catterall *et al* in the *Brit Med J* of 21 June 1975, p.653 *et seq,* and the paper on multiple drug therapy by Price *et al* in the same journal on 5 July 1975, p.10-11.)

6. **(a)** Macrocytosis, anisocytosis and poikilocytosis. **(b) (i)** Serum vitamin B12 and Whole Blood Folate; **(ii)** sternal bone marrow to ascertain whether there is megaloblastic change; **(iii)** test for gastric acid secretion; **(iv)** Schilling test — functional radioisotope test of vitamin B12 metabolism. **(c) (i)** Yes; malnutrition is an important underlying factor in megaloblastic anaemia. Malabsorption could also be a factor. **(ii)** So, too, is pregnancy, especially in the tropics; but less than likely in a 50 year old! **(iii)** Yes. Infestation with a fish tapeworm is a cause of anaemia, particularly in Finland, because the worm ingests vitamin B12 in the alimentary tract of the host — so leaving the host B12 deficient; **(iv)** Yes. Prolonged administration of anticonvulsant drugs may give rise to megaloblastic anaemia.

PLATE 17

1. (a) The calvarium shows multiple well-defined spherical radiolucent areas. **(b)** Multiple myeloma and multiple metastases from primary carcinoma of e.g. lung, breast, thyroid, stomach, prostate. **(c)** The presence of abnormal serum and urinary proteins and of immature plasma cells in the bone marrow would be typical of multiple myeloma. No infective agent has been implicated so that bacteriological and virological examinations would not assist towards a diagnosis. Readers who chose the nonsense in the last option are bamboozled by jargon.

2. (a) The broad square skeletal pattern with hypertelorism and bilateral dentigerous cysts is found in Hunter and Hurler syndromes. While multiple jaw cysts occur in Gorlin syndrome they are odontogenic keratocysts, found in association with basal cell carcinoma and rib defects. The bony lesions of rickets may simulate those of Hurler and Hunter syndromes. In Morquio Ullrich syndrome the facies is not really specific even though the head rests directly on the shoulders. **(b)** In Hunter and Hurler syndromes abnormal accumulations of acid mucopolysaccharide can be demonstrated in cells of inflammatory exudate and of bone marrow, in plasma, and in urine; 'gargoyle' cells characteristic of the recessively inherited disorders of mucopolysaccharides may be found in many body tissues in Hunter and Hurler syndromes. Rickets responds to vitamin D therapy but Hunter, Hurler and Morquio Ullrich do not. Excretion of keratosulphate in urine is a constant feature of Morquio Ullrich syndrome but not of the others in this list.

PLATE 18

1. (a) Thickened skull with loss of distinct inner and outer tables and 'cotton wool' appearance. **(b)** Paget's disease of bone. **(c)** Serum alkaline phosphatase raised to 20-100 K.A. units (normal 3-13 K.A. units). Urinary hydroxyproline also raised. **(d)** At present no curative treatment has been convincingly demonstrated. Calcitonin therapy gives relief of bone pain but it is not yet known whether it prevents deformity from occurring. See leading article, 'Paget's Disease', *British Medical Journal* (1977) 1: 1427-8.

Answers to questions on page 37 (cont.)

2. **(a) (i)** Many unerupted teeth; **(ii)** Wormian bones in skull posteriorly; **(iii)** small maxilla. **(b)** Cleidocranial dysostosis. **(c)** Ascertain presence, absence or partial absence of clavicles. **(d)** Chest X-ray — to determine presence of clavicles; X-ray spine, pelvis and base of skull — to observe any defective bone development. **(e) (i)** Surgical exposure of unerupted permanent teeth and removal of supernumerary teeth; **(ii)** prosthodontic treatment.

Answers to questions on page 39

PLATE 19

1. **(a)** This is hemifacial microsomia which is usually unilateral, never symmetrical, and has no known familial pattern of inheritance. The defects in the mandible may range from stunting of the condyle to complete absence of the ramus and part of the body. **(b)** Early surgical repair is usually followed by poor subsequent growth especially where substantial defects exist in the masticatory muscles on the affected side. **(c)** It arises once in about 4,000 live births.

2. **(a)** Parotid gland. **(b)** Punctate and globular sialectasis. **(c)** Sjogren syndrome and chronic parotitis; the sialographic appearances are not specific. **(d)** In the presence of acute inflammation.

Answers to questions on page 41

PLATE 20

1. **(a)** Bilateral symmetrical expansion of the mandibular angles with multiloculated radiolucent areas. **(b)** Cherubism. **(c)** Yes, as an autosomal dominant trait with variable expressivity. **(d)** None, apart from possibly raised alkaline phosphatase in the active phase of the disease. **(e)** Loose fibrous tissue with multinucleated giant cells scattered diffusely throughout the stroma. **(f)** The prognosis is good. By early adult life the lesions tend to regress and the appearance improves to a varying degree.

2. **(a)** Hypohidrotic ectodermal dysplasia is an X-linked recessive trait, carried by the female and usually manifest in males. Hypodontia and thin hair result from a suppression of

ectodermal elements in the stage of morphodifferentiation. The conical incisors may fail to erupt and the mouth is frequently dry. **(b)** The nails of fingers and toes are spoonshaped, and a starch-iodine test of the skin demonstrates an inability to sweat. The eyelashes and eyebrows are often entirely missing. See also Plate 2 figure 6.

1. **(a)** Parotid sialogram, lateral oblique view. **(b)** Contrast medium is introduced into the duct system. **(c)** The main ducts are distended giving a "sausage-string" appearance. **(d)** It occurs in chronic obstructive sialadenitis.

2. **(a)** Mucous cysts of the antrum are symptomless benign lesions. They may give the radiological appearance of a dentigerous or radicular cyst. **(b)** They are observed in X-rays of about one-third of the young adult population. **(c)** They do not affect the vitality of adjacent teeth. **(d)** They usually disappear spontaneously and require no formal treatment.

1. **(a)** Sickle-shaped red blood cells. **(b)** Sickle cell anaemia. **(c)** Negroes. **(d)** In this condition there is an abnormal haemoglobin (haemoglobin-S) which is much more insoluble in its reduced state. The red cells of a patient with the sickle cell trait may be precipitated into 'sickling' by a state of deoxygenation during a general anaesthetic. Any negroid patient should be screened for this trait before having a general anaesthetic. **(e)** The test consists of placing a drop of the patient's blood on a slide, adding a reducing agent (sodium dithionite) and covering with a cover slip. If positive, sickle cells will be evident on microscopic examination.

2. **(a)** Some small radiopacities in or superimposed on the ascending ramus of the mandible. **(b)** The correct answer is **(iii)**. It is an example of dystrophic calcification, probably post-infective, and involving lymphoid tissue such as tonsil or lymph glands.

Answers to questions on page 47

PLATE 23

1. **(a)** Radiolucent areas. **(b)** In view of the history, primary or secondary hyperparathyroidism must be suspected. **(c) (i)** Biochemical tests of blood and urine for elevated calcium levels; **(ii)** biopsy if swelling of the jaw is also present; **(iii)** radiological survey of the skeleton. Early bone changes can often be demonstrated in phalanges. **(d)** Yes, by removal of hyperplastic or neoplastic parathyroid glands.

2. **(a)** Radiolucent area. **(b)** Secondary tumour, possibly from a bronchial primary. The combination of Cushing's syndrome with osteolytic lesions in bones would suggest ectopic hormone production by a malignant tumour. This is an established feature of some malignant tumours, e.g. of lung, and this site would also account for the recent history of pleurisy. **(c)** The patient should be referred to a general physician for general clinical examination and radiographic investigations to ascertain whether other tumour deposits are present.

Answers to questions on page 49

PLATE 24

1. **(a)** Treacher Collins syndrome (mandibulofacial dysostosis), in which 50% of cases show autosomal dominant transmission. **(b)** Symmetrical antimongoloid sloping of the orbits, abnormalities of the auditory ossicles, deficient malar bones and absent zygomatic arches are invariably found in the radiological examination of these cases.
figure 4.)

2. **(a)** The digital markings produce a 'beaten copper' skull commonly found in Crouzon and Apert syndromes. The cranium is brachycephalic and the maxilla severely hypoplastic. The coronal, sagittal and lambdoidal sutures are synostosed in a majority of cases. **(b)** All may be found because of associated aural atresia, optic nerve damage, maxillary deficiency, epilepsy and cleft palate.